Get Through

MRCPsych Part 1:
Preparation for the OSCEs

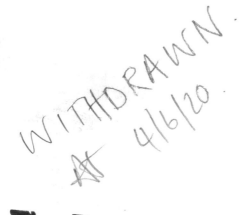

This book is dedicated to my mother Mrs Kosalai Mohana Murthy,
my father Mr Mohana Murthy, my family and
to my respected teachers

Get Through

MRCPsych Part 1:

Preparation for the OSCEs

Sree Prathap Mohana Murthy MB BS (MRCPsych)

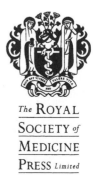

The ROYAL
SOCIETY *of*
MEDICINE
PRESS *Limited*

© 2004 Royal Society of Medicine Press Ltd

Published by the Royal Society of Medicine Press Ltd
1 Wimpole Street, London W1G 0AE, UK
Tel: +44 (0)20 7290 2921
Fax: +44 (0)20 7290 2929
E-mail: publishing@rsm.ac.uk
Website: www.rsmpress.co.uk

British Library Cataloguing in Publication Data
A catalogue record for this book is available from the British Library

ISBN 1-85315-590-X

Distribution in Europe and Rest of World:

Marston Book Services Ltd
PO Box 269
Abingdon
Oxon OX14 4YN, UK
Tel: +44 (0)1235 465500
Fax: +44 (0)1235 465555

Distribution in the USA and Canada:

Royal Society of Medicine Press Ltd
c/o Jamco Distribution Inc
1401 Lakeway Drive
Lewisville, TX 75057, USA
Tel: +1 800 538 1287
Fax: +1 972 353 1303
E-mail: jamco@majors.com

Distribution in Australia and New Zealand:

Elsevier Australia
30–52 Smidmore Street
Marrickville, NSW 2204,
Australia
Tel: + 61 2 9517 8999
Fax: + 61 2 9517 2249
E-mail: service@elsevier.com.au

Phototypeset by Phoenix Photosetting, Chatham, Kent
Printed by Bell and Bain Ltd, Glasgow

Contents

Introduction

The OSCE (objective structured clinical examination) is a test of clinical and communication skills, and was introduced in the MRCPsych part I examinations in Spring 2003.

There are at least twelve stations, each requiring you to undertake a task. There may be additional rest stations, where you either have a rest or perform a pilot task that does not contribute to your overall mark. All stations are compulsory.

You have one minute to carefully read the instructions for each station. These are posted outside the station. A bell will ring when you may enter the station.

Each station lasts seven minutes. There will be an examiner in each station, but for the purposes of the OSCE you should ignore the examiner. You should only direct comments to the examiner if the examiner or the instructions specifically ask you to do so. On entering the station it may be best to acknowledge the presence of the examiner by eye contact, but then turn your attention to the patient and greet them politely.

A bell will ring after **six minutes** and another bell will ring when the **seven minutes** are up. You must then stop the task, go and wait outside the next station. Do not forget to thank the patient and examiner before leaving. Outside the station, do not allow yourself to become distracted by thinking about the station you have just completed – focus on the next station.

Each station consists of a scenario that a competent SHO in **general adult or old age psychiatry** should be expected to deal with. Although you will need to have a certain amount of knowledge to succeed in the OSCE, it is important to realise that the exam is testing your **clinical and communication skills.** You need to be able to use your knowledge in a clinical setting, assessing patients by asking the right questions and reassuring patients appropriately, accurately and sensitively.

Reading textbooks alone will not help you pass the OSCE. You need to polish your interview skills by talking to real patients and ideally your performance should be observed by senior colleagues (registrars or consultants) who can offer constructive criticism.

An OSCE exam needs rigorous practice (in groups please) and an ability to apply your hard earned medical skills in a proper manner. Here your attitude, confidence, and communicating skills will be tested, as well as your knowledge.

About myself

I am training at North Essex Mental Health Partnership NHS Trust in Colchester. I passed my MRCPsych part 1 in Autumn 2003. When I prepared for my OSCE exam, there was no textbook available for OSCE exams in psychiatry.

I collected information from websites, textbooks, course materials, information leaflets and various other sources. I thought that it would be a good idea to put this information into a book to help future candidates. I hope that this book serves its purpose!

Sree Prathap Mohana Murthy

About this book

This book contains those stations/questions that have been encountered by candidates in previous MRCPsych part 1 OSCE exams, and a few others that might be important and are likely to appear in the future examinations. I hope that the book will give an overview of what the OSCE exam is all about. However, reference to standard textbooks is also recommended.

Under each chapter, I have covered most of the questions that you are likely to be asked, and it is impossible to ask all of them in 7 minutes. In practice, different candidates would be asked different questions under the same topic.

Everyone has their own interview style, and this should not change if it works well for you. My advice is to use few words in the interview.

The answers I have given should be used as a guide to form your own responses.

The list of skills to be tested includes:

1. History taking

2. Counselling

3. Clinical examination

4. Procedures

5. Interpretation of blood results

6. Risk assessment

7. Prescribing appropriate treatment

8. Discussion of treatment options

9. Giving an explanation about a disease or a drug

10. Telephone conversation.

The following steps must be followed for all the stations, except those with manikins:

Step 1: Greet and introduce yourself.

Step 2: Purpose of visit should be explained.

Step 3: Obtain permission before you proceed.

Step 4: Build rapport and address the patient's/relative's main concerns.

Step 5: Start with open questions and then proceed to closed questions.

Hints for OSCE

- It is useful and makes sense to practise OSCE in groups. Never read alone.

- Avoid using complicated medical terms unless it is really necessary. Give information to patients in a way they can understand.

- Always introduce yourself to the patient first, and outline what you are going to do in broad terms.

- Listen to the patient. Pick up clues from what the patient says to you.

- Adapt to the situation and be prepared for anything.

- Use appropriate body language.

- Always appear confident, calm and in control of the situation. In short, be professional.

- Respect patients' dignity and privacy and protect confidential information.

- Be honest and trustworthy. Never give false information.

- At the end of each station, thank the patient and the examiner.

SCHIZOPHRENIA

Task: This lady Mrs Bennett, is the divorced mother of one of your patients, Stephen Bennett, who is a 21-year-old university student recovering from a recurrence (second episode) of a schizophrenic illness. This first presented with an acute onset 3 years ago. He stopped medication one year after the first episode and relapsed 6 months ago. Both illnesses were of sudden onset and symptoms included auditory hallucinations and thought withdrawal. His mother is very worried. She has asked to discuss him with you at the outpatient clinic. Her son is willing for you to discuss his case with his mother. Explain the nature of schizophrenia and the long-term prospects for her son.

- Greet and introduce yourself
- Purpose of visit should be explained
- Obtain permission before you proceed
- Build rapport and address the relative's main concerns

What is schizophrenia?

Most people have heard the word 'schizophrenia' but are not really sure what it means. Schizophrenia is a common mental illness which affects one person in a hundred. It usually develops in the late teens or early twenties, although it can start in middle age or even much later in life.

Schizophrenia means that a person finds it difficult to decide what is real and what is not real – it is a bit like having a dream when you are wide awake.

How can it affect an individual?

It can affect an individual's everyday life in many ways, such as:

- A person with schizophrenia may act in an odd or strange way. The person's thinking may be muddled and confused and they may have abnormal experiences. They may have trouble handling everyday problems. They may not be able to concentrate or think clearly. They may find it hard to make conversation or show feelings, which can make it difficult to get on with people.

- Sometimes the person may stop taking care of their basic needs.

Symptoms may be described as positive or negative. These are divided into positive symptoms which are abnormal experiences and negative symptoms which indicate decrease or absence of normal behaviour.

What causes schizophrenia?

No one as yet knows for sure what causes it. There seem to be a number of different causes. Schizophrenia is probably caused by a disturbance in the working of the brain. Since the illness often occurs when the person is under stress, it is thought that stress may act as a trigger.

It is believed that genetic factors provide about half the explanation for the illness. Sometimes, street drugs like cannabis, cocaine, ecstasy, or amphetamines can bring on this illness. It does seem that smoking cannabis can make matters worse in those who already suffer from schizophrenia.

It is not clear what happens when a person develops schizophrenia, but it is thought that chemicals in the brain are affected, resulting in the symptoms of hallucinations, delusions and difficulties thinking.

Can schizophrenia be inherited?

Yes it can. However, this does not mean that if someone in your family has schizophrenia everyone will have it. Nor does it mean that a person with schizophrenia should not marry and have children. It means that if a close relative (e.g. brother, parent or sister) has it, then your chances of getting the illness is higher.

Remember that it is not the illness itself that is inherited, but the tendency to get the illness.

Is schizophrenia a split mind?

There is a common idea that it means having more than one personality or a split personality. This is untrue. People with schizophrenia have only one personality although their personality may be disturbed in some way.

Doesn't schizophrenia make people unpredictable and dangerous?

People who suffer from schizophrenia are rarely dangerous. They are no more unpredictable than anyone else. Despite what is reported in the newspapers people with mental illness and, in particular, schizophrenia are rarely violent but are more likely to be quiet, shy and afraid of what is happening to them.

Any violent behaviour is usually sparked off by street drugs or alcohol. This is the same as for people who do not suffer from schizophrenia.

Can families cause schizophrenia?

In the past, people believed that disturbed parents and families caused schizophrenia. Research has proven that families cannot, and do not, cause schizophrenia.

However, stressful events, or difficult relationships in the family can sometimes trigger an episode of schizophrenia in someone who is otherwise likely to develop it because of genetic and other factors.

How will I know if my relative has schizophrenia?

There is no specific test for schizophrenia. Schizophrenia is diagnosed by doctors when a person displays a specific group of symptoms. Doctors and psychiatrists find out what symptoms are present, from what the patient and their relatives tell them.

What are positive symptoms?

These are the symptoms that individuals experience such as disturbance of thinking process, delusions and hallucinations.

- Disturbance of thinking can occur in different ways, for example, thoughts being put into your head, which seem to come from other people, by telepathy or radiowaves.

- Thoughts leaving your head as if someone is taking them out, so that your mind is blank and you are unable to think about anything.

- Thoughts seeming to be spoken aloud so that everyone knows what you are thinking and none of your thoughts are private.

What are delusions?

A delusion is a false belief which appears to be quite real to the person with schizophrenia, for example:

- Believing that another person has control of your thoughts or actions, and that you are unable to stop them.

- Believing that someone is trying to harm you or kill you for no good reason, or that you are being persecuted.

- Believing that things you see or read about have a special message for you.

- Believing that you are a special person or that you have some special powers.

What are hallucinations?

Hallucinations are false perceptions. This means that the person hears, sees or smells things that cannot be heard, seen or smelt by others. Hearing voices is a very common symptom of schizophrenia. The voices will appear real to the person and may come from the next room or outside. Sometimes they will seem to come from inside a person's head or from a part of their body or, they believe that something or someone is touching them when there is no one there and nothing to explain this.

What are negative symptoms?

These symptoms are usually apparent as changes in a person's behaviour. They are called negative symptoms because they indicate decreases or absences of normal behaviour. For example:

- Lack of motivation to do anything.

- A decrease in all activity levels – ranging from hobbies and leisure pursuits to self-care such as washing.

- Inability to show any emotion; the person may appear flat and may not show any feelings or emotions.

- Inability to enjoy activities that used to give pleasure.

- Disinterest in conversation and talking; the person will not start conversations and will answer with one word, if at all.

These symptoms can be very distressing for relatives. However, it is important to remember that these symptoms are part of the illness and not due to the person's being lazy or hurtful.

Are there any other symptoms?

Yes, there are other symptoms worth mentioning such as language difficulties, odd habits and changed feelings or emotions.

- **Language difficulties:** Sometimes people with schizophrenia will talk in a way that is hard to follow. They may make up words or use odd expressions.

- **Odd habits:** These may include standing or sitting in unusual ways, peculiar mannerisms or habits.

- **Changed feelings or emotions:** Sometimes people with schizophrenia show no feelings or emotions. At other times they may laugh or cry when they are not feeling happy or sad.

What should I do if I think my relative has schizophrenia?

If you think your relative has schizophrenia then you should encourage the person to see his/her GP. If the person is unwilling or refuses to see the GP then you should contact his/her GP and seek advice.

How do you treat this illness?

When a person becomes mentally ill, they are usually treated in the hospital for a further assessment and diagnosis to be made. Afterwards, they can often be treated whilst living at home, especially if they have a supportive family.

Drugs help to alleviate the most disturbing symptoms of the illness. However, they do not provide a complete answer. Support from families and friends, other forms of treatment and services such as supported housing, day care and employment schemes also play a vital role.

What medications are there and how do they work?

There are medications called antipsychotics that help to reduce the symptoms and the anxiety associated with the symptoms. These are made up of chemicals that alter and correct the chemical imbalance in the brain.

Medication is the mainstay of treatment for schizophrenia. We can't cure the illness completely but we can control the symptoms.

Medication works in two ways:

1. It reduces the symptoms of an attack of the illness.

2. Once the symptoms have improved it helps prevent further attacks or the symptoms getting worse.

What will happen if I stop taking my medication? (if the patient asks this question)

If an individual stops taking his/her medication against the advice of their doctor then the chances of their having an attack of schizophrenia are more than doubled. It is, therefore, very important that an individual keeps taking their medication even when they feel completely well.

Is there any medication that has been proven to work?

All antipsychotic medication has a beneficial effect on the symptoms of schizophrenia, but individual patients respond differently to different medication and may need different doses to have the desired effect.

Does the medication have any side effects?

Yes, unfortunately, medication for the treatment of schizophrenia can have unwanted side effects. These are not usually life-threatening, and should be discussed with the doctor or psychiatrist. Some common side effects include drowsiness, shakiness, restlessness, muscle stiffness, increased appetite, weight gain, dry mouth and dizziness, especially when standing up suddenly. Some of the newer medication does not have the unpleasant side effects of restlessness, muscle stiffness, and shakes and is equally effective.

What other treatments would/could be useful?

Several other forms of therapy may be helpful in assisting recovery, in addition to the conventional treatments. Some examples are:

- Relaxation therapy

- Aromatherapy

- Talking therapy

- Exercise

- Family therapy.

Major stressful events such as a death in the family, loss of job or break up of a relationship can make schizophrenia worse or trigger off a relapse of symptoms.

Once a person has been diagnosed with schizophrenia the family and the environment in which they live can contribute in a positive or negative way.

How can I help my relative?

You can help your relative or friend who is suffering from schizophrenia in a number of ways:

1. By encouraging the person to take their medication, especially when they are feeling well.

2. By trying to reduce stressful events or helping the person to cope with stress. Where stressful events cannot be avoided, try and give the person as much notice as possible to introduce change in a gradual way. It is impossible to avoid all stress. However, family members can help one another to cope with difficulties.

3. People can support the individual by encouraging them to regain their former skills. If they nag or criticise the person or push them too hard, it may make things worse. On the other hand if too much is done for them, this can make them worse too. Try not to be too fussy or overprotective. It is very important that the person is encouraged to lead an independent life and gain confidence.

4. Sometimes the person may become depressed and fed up. This is difficult to cope with, but try to be sympathetic and supportive. Don't blame the person; it is NOT their fault. Try to build up their confidence and be encouraging and positive.

5. Living with a person with schizophrenia can be challenging. They may behave in strange ways; stay in bed all day or take hours to get things done. They may seem as though they don't care about anything or anyone. It is hard not to get angry, but this will not help. Try to be patient and encourage gradual change – try not to criticise or punish the person. Encourage the patient and praise their efforts.

How long will he/she have to continue the medication?

The medication controls the symptoms and promotes recovery, but it does not cure the illness. The symptoms often tend to come back. This is much less likely to happen if the person continues taking medication even when they feel well. For most people, the symptoms usually come back in about six months after stopping medication. A small number of people are able to stop medication with no ill effects. Most people, however, need to take maintenance therapy indefinitely, to prevent relapse. For the best outcome, everyone involved, including the person, the family, the community psychiatric team and others need to work together from an early stage.

What is the community psychiatric team?

The community psychiatric team includes doctors, nurses, social workers, psychologists, occupational therapists, physiotherapists and others who have different skills in assessing and enhancing the abilities of the affected person. These include: help in understanding and coping with the condition, rebuilding confidence, providing support, education about the disorder, and counselling.

How effective is treatment? What happens in the long term?

We can't cure schizophrenia. We can only control the symptoms. Some people have only one attack but many people will experience periods when the symptoms return – these are called relapses. A few sufferers will have symptoms all the time.

The illness is likely to affect studies, work and social life. However, many people with schizophrenia live independently, and more and more people are able to work and to have families.

What can I do to help my situation? (if the patient asks this question)

Seek professional advice from your GP and your care coordinator or psychiatrist. There are also voluntary organizations who help and advise patients suffering from schizophrenia, e.g. MIND, National Schizophrenia Fellowship and SANE, whose local contact numbers can be available from the above professional or your local Yellow Pages directory. We will get you an information leaflet on schizophrenia. It has a list of self-help groups, support groups, books and websites with information for patients as well as carers.

Are there any rehabilitation programmes available?

Schizophrenia makes it difficult to deal with the demands of everyday life. Ordinary activities like washing, answering the door, shopping, or making a phone call can seem like huge hurdles. To some extent, drugs help to over-come such problems. However, it is more helpful in the long run if support includes nurses, key workers, occupational therapists and other members of the community mental health team. These provide access to a wide range of services.

After an acute illness, it is often helpful to attend a day unit, starting with physical activities and going through creative pursuits such as painting and pottery to more demanding 'work-like' activities. The idea is to help people get into or back to work. Other services such as unemployment initiatives, and sheltered work, supported accommodation schemes, drop-in centres and day care facilities also play a vital role. For those people whose illness is more prolonged and severe, a specialist rehabilitation service, including residential care may be available.

ELECTROCONVULSIVE THERAPY

Task: Explanation of electroconvulsive therapy to the patient. You are seeing Mr White, a 55-year-old man suffering from a major depressive disorder. He has been treated with two different antidepressants on adequate dosage and for adequate duration (6 weeks) but has not improved. He did comply with these treatments. Your consultant has proposed that he is treated with ECT.

You are asked to give the patient information about ECT with a view of assisting him to decide whether or not he is willing to agree to have ECT. You are not required to assess his capacity to give consent.

- Greet and introduce yourself

- Purpose of visit should be explained

- Obtain permission before you proceed

- Build rapport and address the patient's main concerns first

What does ECT stand for?

ECT stands for electroconvulsive therapy.

Why is ECT used?

Most people who have ECT are suffering from depression. Although we have a variety of different tablets for depression some people do not recover completely and others take a long time. ECT is often used for these patients. In severe cases of depression, ECT may be the best treatment and it can be life-saving.

Why has ECT been recommended for me?

ECT is given for many reasons. It may be very helpful if you did not get better with antidepressant drugs. The other situations where it is very helpful are:

- ECT is most commonly used to treat severe depression not responding to drug treatment.

- It may be helpful if you can't take antidepressant drugs because of the side effects.

- It may help if you have responded well to ECT in the past.

- It may help if you feel so overwhelmed by your depression that it's difficult to function at all, and that your life is in danger because you are not eating (or) drinking enough and wishing to kill yourself.

Is it not a barbaric treatment?

No, not at all. Due to the advances in the field of anaesthesia and with modern equipment, ECT has become more sophisticated and you may not experience any pain or suffering. People show good improvement following ECT treatment.

What will actually happen when I have ECT?

The treatment takes place in a separate room and only takes a few minutes. The anaesthetist will ask you to hold out your hands so you can be given an anaesthetic injection. It will make you go to sleep and cause your muscles to relax completely. You will be given some oxygen to breathe as you go off to sleep. Once you are fast asleep, a small amount of electric current is passed across your head and this causes a mild fit/seizure in the brain. There are little movements of your body because of the relaxant injection that the anaesthetist gives. When you wake up, you will be back in the waiting area and there will be a nurse accompanying you.

What will happen immediately before the treatment?

An ECT treatment involves having an anaesthetic. You will need to fast (have nothing to eat and drink) from about midnight the night before each treatment. This will involve having no breakfast or tea or coffee on the morning that you have ECT.

How will I feel immediately after ECT?

Some people wake up with no side effects at all and simply feel very relaxed. Others may feel somewhat confused or have a headache. There will be a nurse with you when you wake up after the treatments to offer you reassurance and make you feel as comfortable as possible.

How does ECT work?

The exact mechanism is not known.

During ECT, a small amount of electric current is passed across your brain. This current produces a fit/seizure which affects the entire brain including centres which control thinking, mood, appetite and sleep. Repeated treatments alter the chemical imbalance in the brain and bring them back to normal. This helps you begin to recover from your illness.

How well does ECT work?

Over 8 out of 10 depressed patients who receive ECT respond well, making ECT the most effective treatment for severe depression. People who have responded to ECT report themselves to be more optimistic, making them feel like themselves again, less suicidal, and that life is worth living. Most patients recover their ability to work and lead a productive life after their depression has been treated with a course of ECT.

What is a course of ECT?

A course of ECT involves 6 to 8 treatment sessions on an average. ECT is usually given twice a week. It is not possible to say exactly how many treatments you may need. Some people get better with a few treatment sessions but others may need as many as twelve and very occasionally even more.

What are the side effects of ECT?

Some patients may be confused and get headaches just after they awaken from the treatment, and this generally clears up within an hour or so. Sometimes your memory of recent events may be upset and at times simple things, may be temporarily forgotten. In most cases this memory loss goes away within a few days or weeks, although sometimes patients continue to experience memory problems for several months. But ECT does not have any long-term effects on your memory or your intelligence.

Are there any serious risks from the treatments?

ECT is amongst the safest medical treatments given under general anaesthesia; the risk of death or serious injury with ECT is rare and occurs in about one in 50,000 treatments. This is much lower than that reported for childbirth. Very rarely deaths do occur and these are usually because of heart problems. Even when you have heart problems, it may still be possible for you to have ECT safely with special precautions such as heart monitoring. We will ask another specialist to advise if there are grounds for concern.

What other treatments could I have?

Antidepressant drugs may be available to treat your particular condition and it is possible that some of them may work as well as ECT. Psychological or talking treatments are available, but they are useful for milder forms of depression.

Will I have to give my consent? Can I withdraw my consent to have ECT?

At some stage before the treatments, we will ask you to sign a consent form for ECT. If you sign the form it means that you are agreeing to have up to a certain number of treatments (usually 6). You can refuse to have ECT and you may withdraw your consent at any time, even before the first treatment has been given. The consent form is not a legal document and does not commit you to have the treatment. It is a record that an explanation has been given to you and that you understand to your satisfaction what is going to happen to you. Withdrawal of your consent to ECT will not in any way alter your right to continue treatment with the best alternative methods available.

Are there any risks in not having ECT as recommended?

If you choose not to accept your doctor's recommendation to have ECT, you may experience a longer and more severe period of illness and disability than might otherwise have been the case.

What about counselling?

This is generally more useful in milder depressions. Currently, your depression is too severe for you to benefit from them. It is not a good idea to go for counselling at this stage.

What about another drug?

ECT usually works more quickly than medication. But with regard to medication, we could try yet another antidepressant drug. However, you may have to wait for up to 6 to 8 weeks to know whether the new drug is effective, and there is the possibility of new side effects. Drug therapy also has risks and complications and drug treatment is not necessarily safer than ECT.

My friend had ECT in the past. She suffered memory problems and confusion. Can anything be done to reduce it?

We calculate the lowest, efficient dose for each individual patient and give treatment only twice a week, reducing this to once a week if necessary. If there are serious concerns about memory problems, instead of giving the electrical stimulus bilaterally across both temples, we can give it unilaterally to just one side of the head.

What ECT cannot do?

The effects of ECT will only relieve the symptoms of depression, but will not help all your other problems. An episode of depression may produce problems with relationships or problems at home or work. These problems may still be present after your treatment and you may need further help with these. Hopefully, because the symptoms of your depression are better, you will be able to deal with these problems more effectively.

BIPOLAR AFFECTIVE DISORDER

Task: Mrs Smith, a 32-year-old office clerk has recently recovered from her first episode of mania and is awaiting discharge. She wants to talk to you more about the nature of the illness, the aetiology, signs and symptoms, prognosis and the treatment options. She is planning to start a family.

- Greet and introduce yourself
- Purpose of visit should be explained
- Obtain permission before you proceed
- Build rapport and address the patient's main concerns first

Can you tell me more about my diagnosis?

You have been suffering from a manic episode. It is usually a short-lived illness, which, with treatment, you would expect to recover from in a couple of months. However, people who have had a period of mania also suffer from the other side of the illness which is depression. Since it often occurs in the same person, the illness is called manic-depressive illness. It is also called bipolar disorder because there are the two poles of mania and depression.

Can you tell me more about the 'mood swings'?

We all experience minor changes in our mood from one day to the next. We may feel happy or sad. There is usually a good reason for these changes and our mood is appropriate for what is happening in our lives at the time. However, people who have bipolar disorder tend to have major changes in mood for no obvious reason. The mood changes involved in bipolar disorder range from one extreme to another. At one extreme the person may feel excessively happy and excited with a huge increase in energy and activity. This condition is called 'mania'. At the other extreme, the person may be severely depressed with a great loss of interest or energy. These mood swings usually last anywhere from a few weeks to a few months.

How common is bipolar disorder?

Bipolar disorder is quite a common illness. About one person in 100 will develop this disorder at some time in their lives. The disorder usually starts before the age of 30 but may occur at any time in the lifespan. Women and men are equally likely to be affected.

13

How does the doctor know I have bipolar disorder?

There is no specific medical test that can be done to decide whether someone has bipolar disorder. Blood tests, X-rays, or other medical tests cannot detect this disorder. This disorder can only be diagnosed by observing your behaviour and by listening to what you and your family say about your pattern of moods and behaviours.

What causes bipolar disorder?

No one knows exactly what causes this.

Bipolar disorder is probably caused by a number of factors including heredity, brain chemicals, and stress.

Heredity

We know that this disorder can be inherited and runs in families. These findings suggest that there is likely to be some kind of faulty gene or genes in the body. If someone in the family has bipolar disorder, other family members are more likely to develop it than people who do not have a relative with bipolar disorder. However, just because one member of the family has this disorder does not mean that all family members will develop it.

Chemical disturbance

People with this disorder seem to have a chemical imbalance in the brain. It is likely that the faulty gene causes the body to produce the wrong balance of chemicals.

Stress

Stressful life events may increase the chance of developing bipolar disorder among those who are at risk. Stressful events may also make further phases of mania and depression more likely among those who already have this disorder.

What are the symptoms of mania?

In an episode of mania, you may feel:

- Very happy and excited.

- Full of energy, very active.

- Unable or unwilling to sleep.

- Behaving in a bizarre way, recklessly spending your money, less inhibited about your social and sexual behaviour.

- Speaking very quickly and jumping very quickly from one idea to another.

- Full of new and exciting ideas and making plans that are grandiose and unrealistic.

- Making odd decisions on the spur of the moment, sometimes with disastrous consequences.

When someone is in the middle of a manic episode they usually do not realise that there is anything wrong. It is often friends, family or colleagues who first notice that there is a problem. Unfortunately, the sufferer will often object if anyone tries to point this out. And when a sufferer has recovered from one of these episodes, they will often regret the things that they did and said while they were high.

Will I get depressed in the future?

Bipolar disorder usually (but not always) involves episodes of depression. Although you must have had phases of mania before, you can be said to have bipolar disorder; you do not need to have phases of depression to have this disorder. Most people with bipolar disorder do, however, have periods of depression at some point in their lives.

How do you know that I am depressed?

When you are depressed you may experience the following symptoms:

- Feeling sad, and miserable
- Loss of energy and greatly decreased levels of activity
- Loss of pleasure and interest in things that you used to enjoy
- Loss of appetite or weight or interest in sex
- Changes in sleeping behaviour (usually sleeping less and waking early)
- Bleak and pessimistic views of the future
- Thoughts of killing or harming yourself
- Loss of self-confidence.

For more information about the depressive phase, please see the chapter on depression.

What are mixed episodes?

This is a confusing condition for both doctors and patients to recognise. Most often, the episode is recognised as only mania or depression, only later to be recognised as 'mixed'.
   Common symptoms of a mixed episode:

- Many symptoms of both mania and depression.
- Very volatile mood, going from laughter to tears or anger in seconds.

- Sometimes it includes mostly the physical symptoms of mania (increased energy, little need for sleep) and the emotional symptoms of depression (sadness, intense despair).

What will happen in the long run?

It is impossible to make future predictions. Each episode of mania, depression, or mixed phase lasts for a while and then stops. The person usually feels completely well again.

The length of time that a person remains well between episodes of illness varies from one person to the next. Some people may have only two or three episodes of illness and other people may have more episodes of illness. The good news, however, is that with regular medication you can reduce or even prevent further episodes of illness.

How severe is this illness?

The severity of illness differs from one person to another and even in the same person, severity varies from one episode to the next. Some episodes may be so severe that the person needs to spend time in hospital. Other episodes could be very mild and may not need hospital care and with early treatment, the episode of illness is likely to be less severe and hospital admission may be avoided.

How is this illness treated?

Bipolar disorder involves a chemical imbalance in the brain. This disturbance can be treated with medications which are called mood stabilisers. But before that, learning to cope with mood swings is vital, and many people have found that sensible life changes can also help. One of the most commonly used mood stabilisers is lithium and there are also other mood stabilisers. Let me tell you more about lithium.

Lithium is a naturally occurring substance, given as a tablet, which is an effective way of preventing mood swings for many people. It can also strengthen the effect of antidepressants. Treatment with lithium is usually started by a psychiatrist; although once it is stabilised it may be taken over by a GP.

How long will it take to work?
It can take 3 months or longer for lithium to work properly, so you may have to be patient and persistent in taking the tablets when nothing very much seems to be happening.

What are the side effects of lithium?
These can happen in the first few weeks after starting lithium treatment. They can be irritating and unpleasant, but often disappear or get better with time. They may include:

- Feeling thirsty

- Passing more urine than usual

- Blurred vision, dry mouth, bad metallic taste in the mouth

- Slight muscle weakness

- Occasional loose stools

- Fine trembling of the hands

- A feeling of being mildly ill

- Weight gain.

If the level of lithium in your blood is too high you will experience:

- Vomiting, staggering, blurred vision and slurred speech.

If this happens you must contact your doctor immediately.

Do I need any blood tests?

At first you will need blood tests every few weeks to make sure that you have enough lithium in your blood, but not too much. You will need to have these tests for as long as you take lithium, but less often after the first few months. You will also need to have blood tests every few months to make sure that your kidney and thyroid gland is working properly.

Are there any dietary restrictions?

You should eat a well-balanced diet and, especially, drink regular amounts of unsweetened fluids. By doing this you can make sure you have a proper balance of salts in your body. Try to eat regularly and avoid drinking too much tea, coffee or cola. These all contain caffeine – this makes you urinate more than usual and so can upset your lithium levels.

What if I want to become pregnant?

If you become pregnant, it's usually best to stop lithium, but it is essential to ask your doctor about this. There is some evidence to show that during the first three months, women taking lithium may be in some danger of interfering with the baby's development. The risk appears to be low, but it is sufficient for doctors to advise the discontinuation of lithium during the early stages of pregnancy. It is therefore important to tell your doctor if you become pregnant, and it is advisable to discuss the effects of lithium and pregnancy before conception. Further it is advisable not to breastfeed if you need to take lithium.

You may suffer a relapse after childbirth. The chances are about 1 in every 3 women who have suffered from manic depression have a relapse after childbirth. I will be happy to discuss that with you, and if you wish, with your husband also.

What will happen if I stop taking the tablets?

It may be tempting to stop taking the tablets before your doctor recommends, either because of the side effects or because you don't seem to need them any more. This is unwise, bearing in mind how catastrophic the consequences can be of a manic episode. One way of feeling better about continuing with the treatment is to discuss this with your doctor and your family when you are well. You can decide in advance how you want to be treated when you are ill.

How can I help myself with this illness?

- **Learn to recognise the onset of mania or depression.** The switch from normal to manic behaviour often happens in a very short space of time. It is possible to learn to recognise your own early warning signs of illness. You can then seek medical help straight away – quick action can often stop the illness from becoming too severe.

- **Knowledge.** Find out as much as you can about your illness and how you can be helped.

- **Stress.** Avoid stressful situations – we know that these can trigger off a manic or depressive episode. We can't avoid all stress in our life, so it's also helpful to learn how to handle stress better. You can do relaxation training yourself with audiocassette tapes; join a relaxation group or seek advice from a clinical psychologist.

- **Relationships.** Episodes of depression or mania can cause great strain on friends and family – you may find that you have to re-build some relationships after such a time. It's important that you have at least one person that you can rely on and confide in. When you are well you should explain the illness to people who are important to you, so that they know what to expect and understand it.

- **Activities.** It is vital to balance your life between work, leisure and relationships with your family and friends. Make sure that you have enough time to relax and unwind. If you are unemployed, think about taking courses or doing some volunteer work that has nothing to do with mental illness.

What are the chances of me getting another episode of mania or depression?

If you are thinking about the chances of having either an episode of mania or depression in the future, it is about 50/50. It is impossible to make future predictions. But in the longer run most people do have another period of depression or mania.

So should I carry on the treatment?

You should certainly carry on the treatment for a longer period of time and it will need to be reviewed by psychiatrists in outpatients.

What should I do now?

I would recommend you to find out more about manic depression, perhaps by joining an organisation like the Manic Depression Fellowship. I will also give you some information leaflets about bipolar disorder which you can go through when you have time, and come back to me if you have any more queries.

ALZHEIMER'S DISEASE

Task: Mr Spencer White is the son of an 82-year-old (Mr White) who was recently seen in the 'memory clinic'. Mr White lives with his 80-year-old wife. He was referred to the clinic by his GP, and following assessment and further investigations the diagnosis of early Alzheimer's disease was made. Mr Spencer White has made an appointment to see you to discuss his father's condition. Explain the nature, aetiology, signs and symptoms, treatments and likely outcomes of his father's condition.

- Greet and introduce yourself
- Purpose of visit should be explained
- Obtain permission before you proceed
- Build rapport and address the relative's main concerns first

Thank you for seeing me, doctor. Can you tell me exactly what is wrong with my father please?

As you know your family doctor has had concerns about your father's memory. We saw him in the memory clinic. After our assessment, we found that he has definite memory difficulties and we carried out some tests and the results obtained suggest that his memory problems are most likely to be due to a type of dementia called Alzheimer's disease.

What is dementia?

Dementia is the name given to a group of diseases that affect the normal working functions of the brain. Although the causes are largely unknown, the effects are all too familiar: a progressive, irreversible destruction of brain cells that leads to memory loss, confusion, and personality and behaviour changes. Alzheimer's disease is one among them.

What is Alzheimer's disease?

Alzheimer's disease is the commonest type of the dementias. Everyone loses brain cells as they get older. In people with Alzheimer's disease, this process is more severe and rapid than in normal ageing. The parts of the brain that deal with memory are usually affected first. The onset of this illness tends to be gradual.

Loss of short-term memory is usually the first noticeable sign. Patients become increasingly forgetful and slowly other parts of the brain are affected. In the later stages people may develop problems with their speech or undertaking practical tasks.

How common is this condition?

It affects 5% of people over the age of 65. Both males and females are affected. Although it mostly affects people over 65, it can also occur in young people. With younger sufferers, there is often a family history. But in most instances it is not inherited.

What tests have you done to confirm that he has Alzheimer's disease?

Making a definite diagnosis of Alzheimer's disease while the person is still alive is difficult. Only at post-mortem can a diagnosis be confirmed. So a thorough medical and psychiatric assessment is always essential.

- We interviewed your parents to obtain a clear history of his problems and we also assessed his mental state.

- We did a thorough physical and neurological examination, which did not reveal any signs of physical illness.

- We did some blood tests to exclude conditions that can sometimes cause memory loss; these were all normal.

- We referred him to the clinical psychologist who assessed his memory and other brain functions in detail. These tests also showed that your father does have clear problems with memory.

- Finally, we did a CT brain scan which showed some changes in his brain tissue.

What will happen in the early stage?

In the early stages a person with dementia often appears confused and forgetful about things that have just happened. He or she may not remember what they did five minutes ago, or where they are. Long-term memory tends to stay intact and for this reason people with dementia often dwell in the past. Also, in the early stages, concentration and decision-making become difficult.

Mood changes are also frequent. A previously happy person may become irritable or depressed over little things. As the disease progresses, confusion, forgetfulness and mood changes become much more obvious. Those affected may become anxious and aggressive, and may wander aimlessly around the house.

Personal safety is also very much at risk, especially for those who smoke or cook. Even simple things like dressing become difficult. The stress upon carers is enormous, as it becomes difficult to leave someone alone for even a few minutes.

What will happen in the final stages?

In the final stages of the disease, people with dementia need a great deal of help. Often they are unable to recognise even close family and friends.

Communication is frequently a problem: the ability to talk clearly and understand what is being said is often lost. Incontinence is common, and those affected often become bedridden or wheelchair-bound. Because of this, many sufferers finally die from an infection or virus such as pneumonia.

Does that mean he is definitely going to get worse?

Unfortunately, it is a progressive condition. The illness cannot be halted or reversed, ultimately I'm afraid that he will deteriorate.

How long has he got to live?

Most studies have shown people to live for 5–10 years after being diagnosed. However these are only rough and average figures and it really is impossible to make firm predictions in individual patients. What we can assure you at this moment is your father's illness is relatively mild at present and he is in good physical health for his age.

What sort of help can you offer with looking after him?

We can offer him help in various different ways:

- First of all, we will be seeing your father in the 'memory clinic' to monitor his response to the drug treatment.

- We have also arranged for one of our community nurses to visit your parents at their home. Both you and your mother will be able to contact her for advice. If your father needs any urgent medical input, she will contact us and make arrangements for it.

- She will work with our social worker to ensure that your parents receive all the benefits to which they are entitled, and that they are offered appropriate practical help.

What sort of help can social services offer?

1. If your father needs help with personal care, such as washing or dressing, then a HOME CARER can visit to assist him.
2. Social services can arrange for him to attend a day centre to provide him with some company and to allow your mother to have a break.
3. Often outside help in the form of meals on wheels, home help etc. make it possible for people to maintain some independence, dignity and privacy.
4. The local occupational therapists should be able to supply bath equipment, banister rails, a wheelchair, and special seating (if necessary in the future) and these can be obtained through social services.
5. The social services are able to provide short stays of 1–2 weeks in a residential home to provide relatives a short period of respite.

6. If a stage comes where your mother cannot manage to care for your father at home then social services can help to organise **permanent care in a suitable residential or nursing home.**

What about financial and legal arrangements?

As dementia progresses, people become increasingly unable to manage their own affairs. Informal arrangements often exist to get around this problem: a friend or relative collects benefits and pensions. It is important, however, to get legal advice before any major problems arise.

In the early stages of the disease the person with dementia may be competent enough to appoint somebody with Power of Attorney for managing his or her affairs. This can be arranged by a solicitor. However, if the person's mental capacity is too limited for a valid Power of Attorney, it may be necessary to put his or her affairs under the jurisdiction of the Court of Protection.

The following are able to offer help on legal and financial issues: Citizens' Advice Bureau, Mind, Alzheimer's Disease Society's legal advisor, or any solicitor.

Where can I obtain more information about Alzheimer's disease?

The Alzheimer's Disease Society is extremely helpful. They produce various books and leaflets. Your father can join a local self-help group to meet other people in the same position who can provide an invaluable source of practical information. Above all as his main carer, your mother will need help and support and we have invited your mother to join the relatives' support group.

DEPRESSION

Task: Mr Smith, a 30-year-old office clerk has recently recovered from his first episode of major depression and is awaiting discharge. He wants to talk to you more about the nature of the illness, the aetiology, signs and symptoms, prognosis and the treatment options.

- Greet and introduce yourself
- Purpose of visit should be explained
- Obtain permission before you proceed
- Build rapport and address the patient's main concerns first

What is depression?

Most of us feel sad or miserable at times. These feelings may follow a disappointment, losses, or a number of other stressful or unpleasant life events. These feelings of sadness are very common and are experienced by everyone.

We recover quite quickly from our sadness, especially if we have other good things happening in our lives. Some people, however, continue to feel extremely miserable for long periods of time even though there may no longer be a good reason for feeling this way, and may find it difficult to get through the day.

Although there is a tendency to label all our unpleasant feelings as 'depression', there are clearly some people whose depression is much more severe than others. Severe depression that occurs for no obvious reason, or that continues for a long time, at least for a period of two weeks is called 'major depression' or a 'depressive disorder'.

How common is depression?

Depression is a common and treatable illness. Research evidence shows that up to 25% of the population may suffer from this disorder at some time in their lives. Most cases of depression are mild, but about one person in 20 will have a moderate or severe episode. It can affect people from any age group and females are affected more commonly than males.

What are the symptoms of a depressive disorder?

1. Feeling miserable. This misery is present for much of the day but may vary in its intensity. The individual usually looks sad and 'down' and may cry often.

2. Loss of interest or pleasure in usual activities, that you used to enjoy.

3. Loss of appetite with excessive loss of weight.

4. Loss of interest in sex.

5. Loss of energy, and greatly decreased levels of activity.

6. Loss of sleep despite feeling exhausted. Sleep is typically restless and unsatisfying with early morning wakening (1–2 hours earlier than usual).

7. Slowed or inefficient thinking with poor concentration, leading to difficulties sorting out problems or making plans or decisions.

8. Bleak and pessimistic views of the future.

9. Thoughts of killing or harming yourself.

10. Loss of self-confidence.

11. Slowed activity and speech.

Any of these features may serve as a warning signal of depression although many may also occur in disorders other than depression.

What causes depression?

No one knows exactly what causes depression. There is no one cause for depression and it varies greatly from one person to another. Depression seems to run in families. It seems that some people have a set of genes that makes them more likely to develop a depressive disorder.

Another factor in the cause of depression is that depression involves a chemical imbalance in the brain. Although the balance may be right most of the time, at other times the balance may change and the person becomes depressed.

Stressful life events also seem to play a part in the onset or relapse of depression. In vulnerable people these unpleasant and stressful life events may be enough to cause or worsen a depressive illness.

An individual's **personality characteristics** may also be an important factor. Some people have a tendency to view things in a negative way even when they are not depressed. In other words, they may have a depressive personality style. People with this kind of personality style may be at greater risk of developing a depressive disorder.

Another possible cause of depression which should not be overlooked is **physical illness** or **medications**. Certain physical illnesses, other substances of abuse, or other medications such as those for heart or blood pressure conditions, may all cause symptoms of depression.

How can I get help?

If you find that your depression is going on for more than a couple of weeks, that it is getting worse or that it is interfering with your normal activities, you should see your family doctor.

Most people suffering from depression get the help they need from their GP. He or she can work out, with you, what sort of help is going to be most useful. In mild depression, counselling may be all that is needed.

What is counselling?

This is a way of talking over your problems with someone, a counsellor, who is not involved in your daily life. He or she can help by listening and allowing you to talk frankly in a way that it is sometimes difficult to do with family and friends. A counsellor may be able to help you to get a more helpful perspective on your problems. Putting feelings into words can help you to think about them more clearly, and to find practical and constructive ways of overcoming problems.

What is the treatment for moderate and severe depression?

For moderate depression medications such as antidepressants and talking treatments may be needed.

For severe depression, antidepressants are usually necessary before talking treatments can be of help, and it usually needs the help of a specialist, a psychiatrist. Only a small number of people with depression ever need admission to hospital. They tend to have depressions that are life-threatening or are just not getting better.

What will happen if I am left untreated?

If left untreated, depression can be so bad that life may not seem worth living. You may feel like ending the pain by killing yourself. If you find yourself in this situation, you must get help by telling your partner, your friend or relative, a professional or the Samaritans. Feeling like this is a phase that many people with depression go through before they get better – it is important to remember that you will get better.

What are the treatment options available?

Since depression is affected by psychological factors and may involve changes in body chemistry, depression is usually best treated by a combination of medical and psychological or talking treatments. Medical treatments include antidepressant medication, electroconvulsive therapy, and psychological treatments including cognitive and behavioural therapy, and learning how to cope with stress.

Can you tell me briefly about antidepressants and what they are used for?

These drugs will usually relieve depressive symptoms in most people and may help to prevent relapse of the illness.

Antidepressants do not relieve your depression straight away. These drugs take some time to have an effect on your mood. In the first few days the drugs tend to have a calming effect. However, after a week or two of taking the medication regularly, this calming effect gives way to increasing alertness and energy. It may take up to eight weeks before the maximum benefits of anti-depressant medication are noticed. Therefore, you should not expect to notice the benefits from this medicine too quickly and there are a number of different types of antidepressant drugs.

How long do I need to take these medications?

Continue taking the medication for about six months to one year after recovery. Even when you are feeling better it is important to carry on taking the tablets as your GP or psychiatrist advises. If you stop them too soon, this will make it more likely that you will become depressed again. The general rule is that you should carry on taking antidepressants at least for 6 months after your depression has lifted.

What is psychotherapy or talking treatment? Is it the same as counselling?

No it is not the same as counselling. It is much more structured. There are a number of different kinds of psychotherapy or talking treatments that are useful for people who are depressed.

There are three useful forms of psychotherapy:

1. Cognitive therapy

2. Behavioural therapy

3. Interpersonal therapy.

What am I likely to gain from cognitive therapy?

People who are depressed tend to feel as if they are a hopeless failure. Cognitive therapy is a type of talking treatment that aims to help people identify their negative ways of thinking and teach them how to think in a more positive way. People learn that they have some control over what happens to them. They learn to bounce back from failure more effectively and to recognise and take credit for the good things in their lives.

Will they try to change the way I behave in behavioural therapy?

Depressed people lack motivation and they often sit for hours, thinking about their problems. Behavioural therapy aims to identify and change aspects of behaviour that cause or prolong symptoms of depression.

Some forms of behavioural change include activity planning, problem solving, goal planning, and social skills training.

What is interpersonal therapy? Do you mean that I have problems with my personality?
No, not at all. This form of therapy aims to help people resolve one or more of their interpersonal problems that may be causing or prolonging symptoms of depression. For example, interpersonal therapy may target the adjustment to difficult life situations and may help with the resolution of interpersonal disputes (e.g. marital problems or disputes with family members at home (or) with colleagues at work).

How can I help someone who is depressed? (if the relative asks this question)

- It is often difficult to know what to say to someone who is very depressed – it may seem that you can't say anything right because they interpret everything in a very pessimistic way. They may be very worried but unwilling or unable to accept advice. So try to be as **patient** and **understanding** as possible.

- Family and friends often want to know what they can do to help. Family members can help one another to cope with difficulties and stressful life situations.

- Being a **good listener** is very important. **Reassurance** that they will come out the other side is invaluable, though it will usually have to be repeated often as depressed people lack confidence and are prone to worry and doubt.

- Spending time with depressed people, encouraging them not only to talk but take their medications, involve them in activities, keep going to do things are worthwhile.

- Above all, if the depressed person is getting worse and has started to talk of not wanting to live, or even hinting at self-harm, take these statements **seriously** and insist that their doctor is informed. Try to help the person to **accept the treatment**.

POSTNATAL DEPRESSION

Task: You are seeing Ms Turner, a 30-year-old married high school teacher. Your elder sister had a baby boy 2 years ago, followed by a severe PND. It improved with outpatient antidepressant drug treatment for 3–4 months. You are 2 months pregnant now. You are worried that you might also suffer. Address the patient's concerns and allay her anxiety.

- Greet and introduce yourself
- Purpose of visit should be explained
- Obtain permission before you proceed
- Build rapport and address the patient's main concerns first

Can you tell me about postnatal depression?

Postnatal depression (now often called PND) means becoming depressed after having a baby and it is one of the common complications following childbirth. It is like other kinds of depression except that it is brought on by having a baby.

How common is it?

It is quite common, yet often unrecognised. One out of every ten women suffers from PND.

When does it happen?

It usually starts within a month of the delivery but can start up to six months later. It can go on for months, or even years, if untreated.

Is it not the same as baby blues?

PND is a lot different from baby blues. Many women, at least one in two would feel a bit weepy, flat and unsure of themselves on the 3rd or 4th day after having a baby. We call this 'baby blues' or 'maternity blues'.

This soon passes. Many women are weary and a bit disorganised when they get home from hospital, but they usually feel on top of the situation in a week or so. However, if it gets worse or lasts more than two weeks we have to consider PND.

What are the symptoms of PND?

The symptoms of postnatal depression are the same as those experienced in a depressive episode. Symptoms include:

- Depressed mood feeling low, unhappy and tearful
- Exhaustion and loss of energy
- Sleep and appetite disturbance
- Feelings of guilt/incompetence/hopelessness
- Suicidal thoughts, plans, or actions
- Loss of libido
- Anxiety and exaggerated fears concerning the self, the baby or the partner.

The mother may feel irritable towards other children, occasionally to the baby and especially to the partner. She may feel unable to cope with the baby, unable to handle and feed the baby and may feel guilty about it. She may feel anxious and that anxiety may also make the mother concerned about her own health and worry about the baby's health.

What causes PND?

We don't know the exact cause of PND. Probably there isn't a single cause, but a number of different stresses may have the same consequence, or may act together.

We know that among these risk factors are:

1. Previous history of depression (especially PND).

2. Lack of support from the partner and family.

3. Recent stressful life events.

4. An accumulation of misfortunes such as bereavement, the partner losing his job, housing and money problems, etc.

5. The mother's loss of her own mother when a child.

However a woman can suffer from PND when none of these apply and there is no obvious reason at all.

Could it be hormonal?

It seems likely that huge hormone changes take place at the time of giving birth, but this evidence is still lacking. Levels of oestrogen, progesterone and other hormones to do with reproduction, which may also affect emotions, drop suddenly after the baby is born. However, women who do, and who do not, get PND have similar hormone changes.

Would mothers with PND harm the baby?

No, they don't. In fact, many mothers, even those without any mental health problems, can sometimes feel like 'throwing the screaming monster out of the window'. Mothers with PND often worry if they might harm their babies, but they never do.

However, there is another serious mental illness called puerperal psychosis, when there is a risk of the mother harming the baby. In this illness, the mother may be convinced or deluded that the baby is evil and she might harm the baby. But fortunately, this is a much rarer condition, affecting only two out of every 1000 mothers.

What treatments are available?

Since PND is similar to depression, the treatment is also similar.

- Usually, the mother may need only **reassurance, practical support and supportive counselling.** We can assist by organising help with childcare, placing the woman in touch with support organisations and helping the woman to recruit support from family and friends.

- We have **self-help** and **support groups** available locally. They encourage mutual support and advice regarding mothering, childcare and dealing with depression.

- If depression is associated with marital problems, they will have to be tackled through **marital counselling.** Give the woman permission to talk openly about her relationship with her partner and about any disappointments or stresses she may be experiencing with her new role.

- One of the most important aspects of treatment is **educating new fathers.** Educate the partner about postnatal depression and the demands of being a mother. Point out to the partner that the woman is in need of practical and emotional support and deal with specific relationship problems.

- It is also very important to address her **social difficulties,** her needs and provide adequate social support.

- For some, **antidepressant drugs** will be needed. In very severe cases, other drugs and even ECT may be needed.

Can I breastfeed when taking the medication?

Yes. You need not necessarily stop breastfeeding. We can find an antidepressant that does not get into your milk and affect your baby in any way.

What are the chances of me getting PND?

The chance of someone without a history of depression getting a PND is 10–15% and someone who already had one episode of PND getting a second one is higher which is around 20–40%.

Are there any ways to prevent it?

Yes, there are some ways to prevent it. Some of the common strategies of prevention and early intervention include:

1. **Prenatal education** – This education would include information about postnatal depression and this can enhance the couple's ability to recognise postnatal illness and to seek appropriate assistance if required, thereby preventing or minimising serious disability and distress.

2. Encourage the mother to keep in touch with the **GP,** to attend **antenatal classes,** take your partner with you and also to keep in touch with the health visitor.

3. Encourage the importance of regular exercise, rest, sleep, nutritious food; maintaining good relationships with your partner and family is important.

4. Techniques such as relaxation training, confidence building courses and assertiveness training may be useful for preventing the escalation of stress and help them to cope with difficult situations. Some researchers have found that psychoeducation and support programmes can halve the chances of getting a second PND.

5. Additionally, it is also recommended that women take steps to enhance their social network prior to birth if the present social network is inadequate. Advise mothers to arrange for extra support at home for at least two weeks, either friends, family, or professional help.

Can PND in the mother affect the baby?

Research evidence shows that PND adversely affects mothering, bonding mother–infant relationship and the emotional development of the infant. That is why we have to diagnose and treat PND as early as possible.

I will give you some information leaflets about postnatal depression which you can go through when you have time, and I will be happy to discuss this with your husband also.

LITHIUM CARBONATE

Task: Mr White is a 30-year-old gentleman who has just recovered from a manic illness, treated under section. He had a similar manic episode 10 years ago and a depressive episode 4 years ago. Your consultant has suggested he take lithium prophylaxis. Explain to the patient the rationale of taking lithium and the practicalities of lithium therapy.

- Greet and introduce yourself

- Purpose of visit should be explained

- Obtain permission before you proceed

- Build rapport and address the patient's main concerns first

When is lithium used?

Lithium is a mood stabiliser. Lithium is used in treating and controlling mood disorders like depression and mania, especially when they keep coming back. It is also used to increase the effect of antidepressant drugs when these are not working enough on their own. Lithium tends to lead to fewer manic and depressive episodes or to their disappearance. Even if these still occur the mood swings are usually less severe, but it may take several months or even years to control mood swing.

What is lithium?

Lithium is a substance which occurs naturally in food and water. Small amounts can therefore be found in the body. However, this does not mean that it is a natural substance everybody needs, and it is therefore important to note that lithium is not given because people have a deficiency of the substance. Certain minerals have high lithium content and it is from this source that the medication lithium salts are made.

Are there any tests to be done prior to commencement of lithium therapy?

It may be necessary for you to undergo a number of tests to ensure that the medication can be used safely, and these include:

- **Heart function test:** people who have a history of heart disease should not be given lithium.

- **Kidney function test:** An evaluation of how your kidneys function is essential because lithium is eliminated from your body in the urine.

- **Thyroid function test:** A test of the thyroid function is also important because lithium may interfere with the thyroid function and may cause underactivity or overactivity of the thyroid gland. Once on lithium, a thyroid test is recommended every six months.

- **Blood tests:** Once you have begun treatment, it will also be necessary to have regular blood tests (sometimes called 'a lithium level', a 'serum lithium level' or a 'plasma lithium level'). This test is important because it enables the doctor to monitor the amount of lithium in the bloodstream, and therefore ensures that your dosage is both effective and safe.

Doses are adjusted to keep the blood level within the range of 0.4 and 1.0 m mol per litre which is considered to be the appropriate therapeutic range to maximise benefits and minimise side effects.

How long do we need to have blood tests?

Blood tests are needed more often in the early stages of treatment or when your dosage is adjusted. In these circumstances, they may be needed at least once a week. Once serum levels have stabilised, they will be needed only once a month and even less frequently later. As a rough guide, blood tests should be done at least every three months once serum levels have stabilised.

Are there any dietary restrictions to be followed while on lithium?

Making sure that the body is provided with proper amounts of salt and water is a very important part of lithium therapy. Here are a few guidelines:

- **To maintain water balance:** drink at least four to six pints of fluid each day. Avoid excessive amounts of coffee, tea or cola drinks containing caffeine. Caffeine causes water loss and can interfere with lithium therapy.

- **To maintain salt balance:** ensure that your diet contains an average amount of salt. Inform your doctor before you begin any new diets, especially low salt diets. Do not fast while taking lithium.

- **To avoid excessive loss of both water and salt:** take special care to avoid situations where you are likely to sweat heavily, such as too much activity in hot weather, exposure to sauna baths, and heavy exercise.

What are the side effects of lithium therapy?

Like other drugs, lithium may cause adverse effects. Some are relatively mild and occur during the initial adjustment period. These can happen in the first few weeks after starting lithium treatment. They can be irritating and unpleasant, but often disappear or get better with time. Many people taking lithium experience no adverse effects at all.

Some of the early adverse effects may include:

- Feeling thirsty

- Passing more urine than usual

- Blurred vision
- Dry mouth
- Bad metallic taste in the mouth
- Slight muscle weakness
- Occasional loose stools
- Fine trembling of the hands
- A feeling of being mildly ill.

Are there are any long-term side effects?

Some of the long-term side effects are:

1. Excessive weight gain.

2. Changes in kidney functioning which may lead to damage.

3. Thyroid changes: Reduced thyroid activity can cause sleepiness, tiredness, lethargy, slowed thinking, feeling cold, headache, dry skin, constipation, muscle aches, unusual weight gain or conversely increased thyroid activity or hyperactivity.

4. Shaky hands.

5. Skin rash.

However, these side effects can be prevented and controlled by regular blood tests, and monitoring.

Are there any dangerous side effects?

If the level of lithium in your blood is too high, you will experience:

- Persistent diarrhoea
- Severe nausea/vomiting
- Severe hand tremors
- Blurred vision
- Slurred speech
- Lack of co-ordination
- Confusion
- Frequent muscle twitching.

This means the lithium is reaching unacceptable levels within the body, and you need immediate attention to avoid serious poisoning. You have to contact your doctor immediately for advice.

Let your doctor know if you have a high fever, involving excessive sweating or vomiting or diarrhoea. It may be necessary to stop taking lithium temporarily until your physical health has returned to normal.

If I don't feel better after a few days, does this mean the medication isn't working?

No. Lithium does not always work quickly. It can take anything from a few days to several weeks for any noticeable improvement to take place. Although some people feel better as soon as they begin taking lithium, most improve more gradually.

If I am pregnant, can lithium prove harmful?

Yes, at certain stages of the pregnancy. There is some evidence to show that during the first three months, women taking lithium may be in some danger of interfering with the baby's development. The risk appears to be low, but it is sufficient for doctors to advise the discontinuation of lithium during the early stages of pregnancy. It is therefore important to tell your doctor if you become pregnant, and it is advisable to discuss the effects of lithium and pregnancy before conception.

Prospective parents should note that there are no known harmful effects on children whose fathers were taking lithium at the time of conception or earlier; on children of women who had taken lithium before but not during pregnancy.

Is it dangerous to drink while taking lithium?

In most cases, it is safe to drink alcohol in moderation. It is best, however, to check with your doctor when starting treatment.

Does lithium interact with 'over the counter drugs'?

'Over the counter medicine' refers to medicines that are available for purchase from community pharmacies without the presentation of a medical prescription. The sale does however have to be supervised by a registered pharmacist.

Yes, it does interact with certain drugs like ibuprofen. The doses of 1600 mg of ibuprofen per day and above have been shown to raise serum lithium levels. However, the maximum recommended total daily dose of ibuprofen is 1200 mg. Doses greater than this should never be taken without consulting a doctor or pharmacist if you are taking or intend to take the combination of these drugs. It is always a good idea to let the pharmacist know about any other medicines which you are taking, so that they can tell you of any potential problem with drug combinations.

Is lithium addictive?

No. There is no evidence whatsoever to indicate that people taking lithium become physically dependent on the medication. However, some research suggests that some people may experience a recurrence of their original symptoms when they stop taking lithium suddenly. But it is important to remember that people need support to withdraw lithium at their own pace.

Is it safe to drive while taking lithium?

This will vary from person to person. Lithium can impair co-ordination and it is therefore important to take particular care when driving or operating dangerous machinery, and stop if it is clear that you cannot do so safely.

Is it safe to exercise regularly?

It is perfectly safe to exercise regularly provided that you ensure you take in sufficient fluids and salt. It is also advisable to time your lithium dose so it is not taken immediately before vigorous exercise.

How long will it prove necessary to take lithium?

This will vary from person to person. Depending on the course of your condition lithium may prove necessary to prevent episodes of mania or depression for the rest of your life. It is not a cure for manic depression, but a preventive medication.

You should have regular reviews of your lithium treatment to discuss with your doctor whether it is still needed. Psychiatric research shows that a large proportion of lithium users will relapse if lithium is stopped, but it is not possible to tell in advance who will have further severe mood swings and who will not.

If you have been completely free of relapses for three to four years, some doctors may be willing to reduce and stop your lithium for a trial period, under close supervision.

Are there people who should avoid taking lithium?

Yes. People who have a history of heart disease are not advised to take lithium.

Does lithium always work?

No. Some people do not respond to lithium therapy and others cannot tolerate it. Some may respond only partially, and may experience reduced or less severe episodes of depression and mania. It is important therefore that you do not raise your expectations too highly, when commencing treatment. It may take six months to a year to achieve a full effect as a preventive treatment.

Are there other treatments for manic depression?

If someone is particularly susceptible to lithium's unwanted effects, carbamazepine and semisodium valproate can be given as an alternative and these are sometimes given in combination with lithium if the mood swings are only partially controlled.

Are there any precautions to be taken prior to beginning lithium treatment?

Yes. Before beginning lithium therapy, your doctor will need some information that includes your medical history including heart disease, thyroid disease, kidney disease, psoriasis or epilepsy or any history of mental health problems in your family, especially mania or depression.

Also tell your doctor about any medications you are taking, especially diuretic medications (water pills used to treat high blood pressure), drugs used for asthma, painkillers, steroids and antidepressants.

Some practical tips when taking lithium

- **Do** ensure that your diet includes plenty of salt and water. A reduction in either may allow lithium to build up to dangerous levels.

- **Do** inform your doctor immediately about any adverse effects you notice. Minor adverse effects can be discussed at routine sessions with your doctor, but any adverse effects mentioned previously should be reported immediately.

- **Do** ensure that you tell any other doctor who is treating you that you are taking lithium, or any other medication. If you are admitted to hospital for any reason, you should also tell the doctor treating you that you are taking lithium. If you are given a lithium treatment card, always remember to take this with you.

- **Don't** double up a dose of lithium if you forget a prescribed dose. If you have missed your regular time by three hours or less, take your normal dose. If you have missed your normal dose by over three hours, skip the forgotten dose and resume your lithium medication at the next scheduled time.

- **Don't** change your prescribed dosage without consulting your doctor. The appropriate dosage will vary from patient to patient and your doctor will be in the best position to judge how much you should take.

CLOZAPINE

Task: Mr Taylor is a 45-year-old gentleman with a diagnosis of chronic schizophrenia resistant to treatment, and he has been on various combinations of medications without much benefit. Your consultant has suggested that he should be started on clozapine. Explain how you would commence him on clozapine and discuss the potential benefits and side effects of clozapine.

- Greet and introduce yourself
- Purpose of visit should be explained
- Obtain permission before you proceed
- Build rapport and address the patient's main concerns first

For what is clozapine used?

Clozapine is one of the newer 'antipsychotic' drugs used to treat symptoms of schizophrenia in people who have not done well on at least two other similar drugs, e.g. who have not responded or who have had unpleasant side effects.

How does clozapine work?

There are many naturally occurring chemical messengers ('neurotransmitters') in the brain and dopamine is one of them. Dopamine is the chemical messenger mainly involved with thinking, emotions, and behaviour. In schizophrenia, it may be overactive which helps to produce some of the symptoms of the illness. The main effect that clozapine has is to block some of the dopamine in the brain, reducing the effect of having high levels, and reducing the symptoms caused by too much dopamine.

Will I need a blood test?

Clozapine can upset the blood of about two or three in every hundred people taking it. It can reduce the number of white cells or neutrophils in the blood (neutropenia). This makes it much harder for your body to fight infections. You must, therefore, have regular blood tests for as long as you are taking this medicine.

How often are these blood tests done?

You will need a test before you start clozapine, then every week for the first 18 weeks, and every two weeks from then on. If you have been taking clozapine regularly for a year without any blood problems, it may be possible to change the blood tests to every four weeks. The blood is usually posted to the CPMS (Clozapine Patient Monitoring Service), who return the results to the pharmacy and doctor.

You may also need extra blood tests if it is thought that your blood is being affected. You must not miss these tests. Your doctor and pharmacist will not be able to let you have any more tablets if you do.

Remember the rule: no blood, no tablets.

When should I take clozapine?

Take your clozapine as directed by your doctor. Try to take it at regular times each day. Taking it at mealtimes may make it easier to remember, as there is no problem in taking clozapine with or after food. If the instructions say to take it once a day, this should usually be at bedtime, as it may make you feel drowsy when first taking it, although clozapine is not a sleeping tablet.

How long will clozapine take to work?

Some effects of clozapine, such as drowsiness, appear soon after taking it. The most important action, helping to control the symptoms of your illness, may take several months or even up to a year of regular medication to become fully effective. In the same way, if your dose or treatment is changed, it may take an equally long time before you notice the effects of such a change.

For how long will I need to keep taking it?

This is very difficult to tell, as people's responses are different. However, you will probably need to continue your treatment for several years. Long-term treatment should be reviewed every three to six months or sooner if there are problems. It is likely that you will benefit from clozapine by taking it for many years.

Is clozapine addictive?

Clozapine is not addictive. There is no evidence whatsoever to indicate that people taking clozapine become physically dependent on the medication.

Can I stop taking clozapine suddenly?

It is unwise to stop taking clozapine suddenly, even if you feel better. Your symptoms can return if treatment is stopped too early. This may occur some weeks or even many months after the drug has been stopped and we call it 'rebound psychosis'.

What should I do if I forget to take it?

Start again as soon as you remember unless it is almost time for your next dose, then goes on as before. Do not try to catch up by taking two or more doses at once, as you may experience more side effects. If you have problems remembering your doses (as many people do) tell your pharmacist, doctor, or nurse about this. There are special packs, boxes, and devices available that can be used to help you remember.

What sort of side effects might occur?

Like other drugs, clozapine may cause adverse effects. Some are relatively mild and occur during the initial adjustment period. These can happen in the first few weeks after starting the treatment. They can be irritating and unpleasant, but often disappear or get better with time. Some people taking clozapine may experience no adverse effects at all. Some of the common side effects are:

Common side effect	What happens
Drowsiness	Feeling sleepy or sluggish
Constipation	Difficulty in passing a motion
Hypersalivation	Your mouth is full of saliva and you may drool
Hypotension	Low blood pressure – this can make you feel dizzy
Weight gain	Eating more and putting on weight
Fever	Rise in body temperature
Palpitations	A rapid heart beat

Are there any dangerous side effects?

One of the more serious side effects is that it can reduce the number of white cells or neutrophils in the blood, resulting in a condition called neutropenia. This makes it much harder for your body to fight infections. On higher dosage, it can also induce a seizure or a fit.

Warning signs: If you think you have a cold, sore throat or any other infection, tell your doctor or nurse immediately. They will arrange a blood test to check your white cell count. If your white cell count is normal you should be able to continue with your treatment, but your doctor will tell you if this is the case.

Will clozapine make me drowsy?

Clozapine may make you feel drowsy or sleepy. You should not drive or operate machinery until you know how it affects you. You should take extra care, as it may affect your reaction times or reflexes. Clozapine is not, however, a sleeping tablet, although if you take it at night it may help you to sleep.

Will clozapine cause weight gain?

When you start taking clozapine, you may experience weight gain. This tends to stop after a time, but can be a problem with clozapine. It is thought that the drug causes an increase in appetite, which then makes you eat more and put on weight. If you do start to put on weight, or have problems with your weight, you should tell your doctor. He/she may be able to change your clozapine dose to reduce this effect. Your doctor can also arrange for you to see a dietician for advice. Any weight you put on can be controlled while you are still taking this drug, with expert advice about diet. Make sure your doctor knows about this if it causes you distress.

Will clozapine affect my sex life?

Drugs can affect desire (libido), arousal (erection), and orgasmic ability. Unlike many other antipsychotic drugs, clozapine has not been reported as having a major adverse effect on the three stages, except by causing drowsiness. However, if this happens, you should discuss it with your doctor, who may recommend a change in dose to help minimise the problem.

Can I drink alcohol while I am taking clozapine?

You should avoid alcohol while taking clozapine, as it may make you feel more sleepy. This is particularly important if you need to drive or operate machinery. You must seek advice on this.

Are there any foods or drinks that I should avoid?

You should have no problems with any food or drink other than alcohol.

Will it affect my other medication?

You should have no problems if you take other medications, although some have been recorded. Clozapine should not be taken with some antibiotics, e.g. co-trimoxazole and chloramphenicol. It can also interact with a few other drugs, including some drugs for depression and some anticonvulsants, e.g. carbamazepine. This does not necessarily mean the drugs cannot be used together, just that you may need to follow your doctor's instructions very carefully. Make sure your doctor knows about all the medicines you are taking. You should tell your doctor before starting or stopping these or any other drugs.

If I am taking a contraceptive pill, will this be affected? (female patients)

It is not thought that the contraceptive pill is affected by clozapine. With many drugs of this type, a woman's periods may be irregular or even disappear. This is less likely with clozapine and so they may reappear or become more regular if changing to clozapine.

Can I drive while I am taking clozapine?

Clozapine can affect your driving in two ways. Firstly, you may feel drowsy and/or suffer from blurred vision when starting to take the drug. Secondly, clozapine can slow down your reactions or reflexes. This is especially true if you also have a dry mouth, blurred vision, or constipation (the so-called 'anticholinergic' side effects). Until these effects wear off, or you know how your clozapine affects you, do not drive or operate machinery. It is advisable to let your insurance company know if you are taking clozapine. If you do not and you have an accident, it could affect your insurance cover.

Who organises the blood monitoring?

The Clozapine Patient Monitoring Service (CPMS) organises the monitoring. This service was set up in 1990. Its main aim is to make sure patients being treated with clozapine are regularly monitored to reduce the risk of any adverse effects on their white cell levels. This way they can alert your doctor quickly if there is a problem. This service keeps track of the progress of every single patient taking clozapine and keeps up-to-the-minute records of all blood tests results.

What form does monitoring take?

Before clozapine is started, a blood test is carried out to check that your white cell count is satisfactory. Then, if all is well, your doctor will start treatment. When treatment starts you will be monitored. This may mean staying in hospital from several days to three–four weeks.

Regular blood testing is the main form of monitoring. You will have a blood test every week for at least 18 weeks. After 18 weeks all your blood results will be reviewed, and if all is well, testing may change to every second week until the end of the first year of treatment.

The risk of neutropenia decreases after the first year of treatment. So if your blood tests have been satisfactory, you should be able to transfer to testing every four weeks. Testing will then continue every four weeks for as long as you are taking clozapine.

What happens if you miss a blood test?

Because of the risk of neutropenia, there is one very important rule about taking clozapine tablets – no blood result, no drug treatment.

How will you start my treatment?

When we want to start anyone on clozapine treatment we have to register the patient. Once you are registered, treatment can begin.

As with other antipsychotic medicines, clozapine can cause some general side effects. To keep these unwanted effects to a minimum, we will start you

43

on a low dose and increase it slowly as well as adjusting the dose depending on how you react. This way of tailoring medicines to an individual is called titration. The aim of titrating clozapine in this way is to achieve the best effect with the minimum of unwanted side effects at the lowest effective dose.

Normally, we will start you on 12.5 mg once or twice on the first day. On the second day you will have one or two 25 mg tablets. If necessary, the daily dose can be increased further by 50 to 100 mg, usually in half-weekly or weekly intervals, up to a maximum of 900 mg per day.

How long will it take before the medicine begins to work and does it work for everyone?

Some people feel the benefit of their treatment within a few days while other people can wait from a few months to a year. Therefore, it's important to be patient and give your treatment a chance to work.

About 6 out of 10 people will benefit from taking clozapine. Some do very well and others will be a bit better. Unfortunately, some people do not respond to the medicine, but they will not be made any worse by trying it.

How will I know the medicine is working?

You will probably find that your relatives, friends or carer notice the reduction in your symptoms before you. You may notice that you feel better and are becoming less withdrawn and able to be more involved in life around you.

How long the medicine should be taken for?

Clozapine should continue to be taken every day as prescribed for as long as you are benefiting from taking it. Treatment should not be stopped because your symptoms have diminished or disappeared. If you stop taking clozapine the symptoms are quite likely to come back.

Just like any prescribed medicine you must be seen regularly by your doctors. If your doctor feels you should stop taking clozapine, for reasons other than neutropenia, withdrawal from the drug should be done slowly over a period of time.

What happens if I miss one dose?

If you miss a dose take your next dose at the normal time. Do not try to make up the missed dose by taking more. Do not double dose.

What happens if I miss more than one dose?

If you have missed more than 48 hours of your medicine, you must contact your nurse or doctor immediately. You must not carry on with the same dose as before. It is essential to start again from 12.5 mg once or twice on the first day under the supervision of your doctor. However, if you tolerated the initial doses of clozapine well, your doctor may be able to increase the dose to your maintenance level more quickly.

Pregnancy and breastfeeding (women)

The safety of clozapine during pregnancy is not clear and therefore should not be taken. Clozapine is also thought to get through to breast milk and so mothers taking clozapine should not breastfeed their babies.

SELECTIVE SEROTONIN RE-UPTAKE INHIBITORS

Task: You have seen Mr Hughes in the outpatients' clinic and he has been diagnosed as suffering from depression. You are planning to start him on paroxetine (SSRI). Explain to the patient about the drug and address his concerns.

Note: The following questions and answers can be used for any of the SSRIs.

- Greet and introduce yourself
- Purpose of visit should be explained
- Obtain permission before you proceed
- Build rapport and address the patient's main concerns first

What are SSRIs?

SSRIs are selective serotonin re-uptake inhibitors.

What is paroxetine?

Paroxetine is one of the SSRIs which belong to a class of antidepressants.

What are SSRIs used for?

SSRIs are antidepressants that are used to help improve mood in people who are feeling low or depressed. All these drugs are sometimes used to help other illnesses, e.g. anxiety, bulimia nervosa, panic attacks, and obsessive-compulsive disorder.

SSRIs are now one of the most commonly prescribed antidepressants, but there are many other similar drugs. All these antidepressants seem to be equally effective at the proper dose, but have different side effects from each other. SSRIs generally have fewer side effects than the older drugs. If one drug does not suit you, it may be possible to try another.

How do SSRIs work?

The brain has many naturally occurring chemical messengers. One of these is called serotonin and this is important in the areas of the brain that control mood and thinking. It is known that serotonin is not as effective or active as normal when someone is feeling depressed. SSRI antidepressants increase the amount of the serotonin chemical messenger and this can help to correct the lack of action of serotonin and improve mood.

When should I take them?

Take your medication as directed by your doctor. If you are told to take your dose once a day this will usually be better in the morning. If you feel sick when first taking the SSRI, this should only last for a few days, but the nausea can be relieved by taking the medication with or after food. Also, taking the SSRI at mealtimes may be easier to remember, and there are no problems about taking any of these drugs with or after food. However, they are not sleeping tablets.

How long will they take to work?

It may take two weeks or more before the SSRIs start to have any effect on your mood, and a further three or four weeks for this effect to reach its maximum. If it has not started working in about six weeks, it is unlikely to work. Unfortunately, in some people, the effect may take even longer, e.g. several months, especially if you are older.

For how long will I need to keep taking these tablets?

This is very difficult to say as people's responses are different. To help you make a decision, it may be useful for you to know that research has shown that:

- For a first episode of major depression, your chances of becoming depressed again are much lower if you keep taking the antidepressant for six months after you have recovered (longer if you have risk factors for becoming depressed again).

- For a second episode, your chances of becoming depressed again are lower if you keep taking the antidepressant for one or two years after you have recovered.

- For depression that keeps returning, continuing to take an antidepressant has been shown to have a protective effect for at least five years.

When the time comes, your doctor should withdraw the drug slowly, e.g. by reducing the dose gradually every few weeks.

Are SSRIs addictive?

SSRIs are not addictive, but if you have taken them for eight weeks or more, you may experience some mild 'discontinuation' effects if you stop taking them suddenly. These do not mean that the antidepressant is addictive but these are more of an 'adjustment' reaction from sudden removal of the drug rather than withdrawal.

Can I stop taking them suddenly?

It is unwise to stop taking it suddenly, even if you feel better. Two things could happen. Firstly, your depression can return if treatment is stopped too early. Secondly, you may experience some mild 'discontinuation' symptoms

What are 'discontinuation symptoms'?

These could include: dizziness, vertigo/light-headedness, nausea, fatigue, headache, 'electric shocks in the head', insomnia, agitation, and anxiety. These can start shortly after stopping or reducing doses, are usually short-lived, will go if the antidepressant is started again, and can even occur with missed doses. These effects have been reported for all the SSRIs, but seem to occur more often with paroxetine than the others.

What should I do if I forget to take a dose?

Start again as soon as you remember, unless it is almost time for your next dose, then go on as before. Do not try to catch up by taking two or more doses at once, as you may experience more side effects. You should tell your doctor about this at your next appointment.

If you have problems remembering your doses (as many people do) ask your pharmacist, doctor, or nurse about this. There are special packs, boxes, and devices available that can be used to help you remember.

What sort of side effects might occur?

Like other drugs, these drugs may cause adverse effects. Some are relatively mild and occur during the initial adjustment period. These can happen in the first few weeks after starting the treatment. They can be unpleasant but often disappear or get better with time. Some of the common side effects are:

Side effect	What happens
Common	
Nausea and vomiting	Feeling sick and being sick
Insomnia	Not being able to fall asleep at night
Sexual dysfunction	Finding it hard to have an orgasm. No desire for sex
Less common	
Restlessness or anxiety	Tense and nervous, and you may sweat more
Headache	Your head is pounding and painful
Loss of appetite	Not feeling hungry. You may lose weight
Diarrhoea	Passing loose, watery stools

Will the drugs make me drowsy?

These drugs may make you feel drowsy, although this effect is less compared with other antidepressants. You should not drive or operate machinery until you know how they affect you. You should take extra care, as they may affect your reaction times or reflexes.

Will the drugs cause me to put on weight?

The other drugs in this group tend to have less effect on body weight. However, if you do start to have problems with your weight tell your doctor at your next appointment, who can then arrange for you to see a dietician for advice. It may be that in the long-term (i.e. over a year or more), there is a tendency to gain a little weight.

Will the drugs affect my sex life?

Drugs can affect desire (libido), arousal (erection), and orgasmic ability. The SSRIs are known to affect all three stages in some people. Delayed orgasm is known to occur in many people. Indeed some of these drugs are now widely used to help treat premature ejaculation. If this does seem to be happening, you should discuss it with your doctor, as a change in drug dose or the time when you take the dose may help to reduce problems.

Can I drink alcohol while I am taking the SSRI?

You should avoid alcohol except in moderation while taking these drugs as they may make you feel sleepier. This is particularly important if you need to drive or operate machinery, and you must seek advice on this.

Are there any foods or drinks that I should avoid?

You should have no problems with any food or drink other than alcohol.

Will the SSRI affect my other medication?

You should have no problems if you take other medications, although a few can occur. The SSRIs can 'interact' with other antidepressants and blood thinners, e.g. warfarin. This does not necessarily mean that the drugs cannot be used together, but you may need to follow your doctor's instructions very carefully. Make sure your doctor knows about all the medicines you are taking. You should tell your doctor before starting or stopping these, or any other drugs.

If I am taking a contraceptive pill, will this be affected?

It is not thought that the contraceptive pill is affected by any of these drugs.

Will I need a blood test?

You will not need a blood test to check on your SSRI.

Can I drive while I am taking the SSRI?

You may feel drowsy at first when taking any of these drugs. Until this wears off, or you know how the drug affects you, do not drive or operate machinery. You should take extra care, as they may affect your reaction times.

It is an offence to drive, attempt to drive, or to be in charge of a vehicle when unfit through drugs. It is advisable to let your insurance company know if you are taking these drugs. If you do not and you have an accident, it could affect your insurance cover.

ATYPICAL ANTIPSYCHOTICS

Task: Mr Williams is a 30-year-old gentleman admitted to the psychiatric ward with a diagnosis of paranoid schizophrenia. He is sensitive to conventional antipsychotics and develops extrapyramidal side effects. Your consultant has decided to start him on an atypical antipsychotic, preferably olanzapine. Explain to the patient about the drug and address his concerns.

Note: The following questions and answers can be used for any of the atypical antipsychotics.

- Greet and introduce yourself

- Purpose of visit should be explained

- Obtain permission before you proceed

- Build rapport and address the patient's main concerns first

What are atypical antipsychotics used for?

These drugs are generally used to help treat illnesses or conditions, such as psychosis and schizophrenia. These drugs seem to be equally effective at the proper dose, but have fewer side effects than the older drugs.

How do they work?

There is a naturally occurring chemical in the brain called dopamine. Dopamine is the chemical messenger mainly involved with thinking, emotions, behaviour, and perception. In some people, dopamine may be overactive and upset the normal balance of chemicals. Excess dopamine helps to produce some of the symptoms of the illness. The main effect of these drugs is to block some dopamine receptors in the brain, reducing the effect of having too much dopamine, and correcting the imbalance. This reduces the symptoms caused by having too much dopamine.

When should I take them?

Take your medication as directed by the doctor. Try to take them at regular times each day. Taking them at mealtimes may make it easier for you to remember, as there is no problem about taking any of these drugs with or after food. If the instructions say to take them once a day, this is usually better at bedtime, as they may make you drowsy at first, but they are not sleeping tablets.

How long will they take to work?

Some of the effects of these drugs appear soon after taking them, for example, the drowsiness. The most important action, to help the symptoms of your illness, may take weeks, or even months of regular medication to become fully effective. Similarly, if your dose or treatment is changed, it may take an equally long period of time before you notice the effects of such a change.

For how long will I need to keep taking them?

This is quite difficult to say at this moment as people's responses are different. You will probably need to continue your treatment for a long time, possibly several years after your symptoms have disappeared, to make sure you have fully recovered from your illness. Long-term treatment should be reviewed at regular intervals, for example, every three to six months or even sooner if there are problems.

Are they addictive?

These drugs are not really addictive. If you have taken them for a long time, you may experience some mild effects if you stop taking them suddenly. The main problem would be your symptoms returning.

Can I stop taking them suddenly?

It is unwise to stop taking them suddenly, even if you feel better. Your symptoms can return if treatment is stopped too early. This may occur some weeks or even many months after the drug has been stopped. When the time comes, we will usually withdraw the drug by a gradual reduction in the dose taken over a period of several weeks.

What sort of side effects might occur?

Like other drugs, these drugs may cause adverse effects. Some are relatively mild and occur during the initial adjustment period. These can happen in the first few weeks after starting the treatment. They can be unpleasant but often disappear or get better with time. Some of the common side effects are:

Side effect	What happens
Drowsiness	Feeling sleepy or sluggish
Dry mouth	Not much saliva or spit
Constipation	You cannot pass a motion
Hypotension	Low blood pressure – this can make you feel dizzy
Weight gain	Eating more and putting on weight

The good thing is that these newer medications do not have the unpleasant side effects of restlessness, muscle stiffness, and shakes but they are equally effective.

Will they make me drowsy?

These drugs may make you feel drowsy or sleepy. You should not drive (see below) or operate machinery until you know how they affect you. You should take extra care, as they may affect your reaction times or reflexes. However, they are not sleeping tablets, although if you take them at night they may help you to sleep.

Will they cause weight gain?

Weight gain with these drugs is quite possible and more likely with olanzapine. In the people who gain weight, most is gained during the first 6–12 months of treatment. It then tends to level out. It is not possible to say what the effect on your own weight may be because each person will be affected differently. If you do start to put on weight or have other problems, you should tell your doctor. He/she may be able to adjust your drug or the dose of your drug to reduce this effect. Your doctor can also arrange for you to see a dietician for advice. If you do gain weight, it is possible to lose it while you are still taking this medication, with expert advice about diet.

Will it affect my sex life?

Drugs can affect desire (libido), arousal (erection), and orgasmic ability. These drugs are not thought to have a significant effect on any of these stages, but problems have been reported occasionally with these drugs. If this happens, however, you should discuss it with your doctor, as a change in dose or drug may help to minimise the problem.

Can I drink alcohol while I am taking these drugs?

If you drink alcohol while taking these drugs it may make you feel sleepier. This is particularly important if you need to drive or operate machinery, and you must seek advice on this.

Are there any foods or drinks that I should avoid?

You should have no problems with any food or drink other than alcohol.

Will they affect my other medication?

You should have no problems if you take other medications, although a few problems can occur. Sedative drugs might make you feel sleepier. This does not necessarily mean the drugs cannot be used together, just that you may need to follow your doctor's instructions very carefully. You should tell your doctor before starting or stopping these, or any other drugs. Make sure your doctor knows about all the medicines you are taking.

What should I do if I forget to take them?

Start again as soon as you remember, unless it is nearly time for your next dose, then take the next dose as normal. Do not try to catch up by taking two or more doses at once, as you may experience more side effects. If you have problems remembering your doses (as many people do) ask your pharmacist, doctor, or nurse about this. There are some special packs, boxes, and devices available that can be used to help you remember.

If I were to take a contraceptive pill, will this be affected? (female patients)

It is not thought that 'the pill' is affected by any of these drugs.

Will I need a blood test?

Not usually.

Can I drive when I am on this drug?

These drugs can affect your driving, e.g. you may feel drowsy. Until this wears off or you know how your drug affects you, do not drive or operate machinery. You should take extra care, as they may affect your reaction times or reflexes, even though you feel well.

It is an offence to drive, attempt to drive, or to be in charge of a vehicle when unfit through drugs. It is advisable to let your insurance company know if you are taking these drugs. If you do not and you have an accident, it could affect your insurance cover.

ANTIDEMENTIA DRUGS – EXPLAIN TO A CARER

Task: Mr Bateman, a 78-year-old gentleman, is diagnosed as suffering from mild Alzheimer's disease. The consultant has decided to start him on donepezil (Aricept). His daughter who is also his main carer has heard that there are new drug treatments available. She has fixed an appointment to see you to discuss more about these drugs.

- Greet and introduce yourself
- Purpose of visit should be explained
- Obtain permission before you proceed
- Build rapport and address the relative's main concerns first

New drugs for dementia

I have heard that there are new drug treatments available for Alzheimer's disease. Could you tell me more about them please?

Yes. You are right. Recently some new drugs have been made available for the treatment of mild to moderate Alzheimer's disease. These drugs are collectively called antidementia drugs or anticholinesterases. There are no major differences between these drugs. Some of the examples include donepezil (Aricept), rivastigmine and galantamine. More drugs are on the way.

How will this Aricept help my father?

It will not cure him completely, but it may help to stabilise the illness or improve it for a while. It may help his memory. He can also have general benefits including improving alertness and motivation. More often carers see general improvements in behaviour or mood.

How effective are these drugs?

Research studies have shown that 50–60% of people who have taken these drugs have shown some improvement or stabilisation of their condition over a period of six months.

How do they work?

In Alzheimer's disease, one of the chemicals in the brain called acetylcholine, which is important for learning and memory, is in short supply. So if you have less acetylcholine activity, then you may have less memory ability and reduced learning. The drugs act by increasing the brain levels of acetylcholine and help to stabilise or improve memory, learning and functioning.

How do we go about starting the drug?

1. First of all, he will be seen in the memory clinic by the specialist.

2. Once the diagnosis is made, then the specialist should initiate the treatment. But before that, we have to find out if the drug suits him.

3. We will take a history, including a detailed medical history to rule out severe heart, kidney or liver problems or breathing problems.

4. Then we will also do a formal assessment of his daily living skills and if all goes well then we may start him on these drugs (like in your father's case).

How is the treatment given?

We will start with one tablet of 5 mg of donepezil (Aricept) once a day. We will need to re-evaluate this dose in about 4 weeks. We shall ask a nurse to see your father after about 2 weeks of treatment to make sure that he is not having side effects.

How long do these drugs take to work?

These drugs take at least 4 weeks to show their full effect at the starting dose. After 4 weeks, we may increase his dose.

How long would he stay on this drug for?

Initially we usually prescribe these drugs for a trial period of 3 months to see, if at the end of 3 months, your father has shown any benefits from this drug. If not we may take him off the drug.

If he does show improvement, then we will need to review him approximately every 6 months to see if it is worthwhile continuing the treatment.

People are often given a screening memory test called the 'mini mental state examination' also called as MMSE. The total score is 30, and we suggest stopping these drugs when the MMSE score goes below 12 out of 30.

However, in some patients, if we stop the drug they may deteriorate rapidly and we may have to consider reintroducing it.

What sort of side effects may occur?

The most common problem is feeling nauseous or a bit sick in the beginning. Therefore we recommend taking the drug with food.

Other common side effects are loss of appetite, tiredness, muscle cramps and sometimes poor sleep.

The uncommon and rare side effects are urinary retention and seizures.

Will these drugs make him feel drowsy?

Drowsiness is not a main side effect of these drugs but if you do feel drowsy, then you should not drive or operate dangerous machinery. You should take extra care as they may affect your reaction times.

Will these drugs cause weight gain?

Weight gain is not a reported side effect of these drugs. But if it happens, tell your doctor at your next appointment.

Can he drink alcohol while he is taking these drugs?

There are no known problems.

Are there any diet restrictions?

You should have no problems with your food or drink.

Will these drugs affect his other medication?

You should have no problems if you take other medications.

Will he need a blood test?

You should not need to have a blood test to check on your drug, although your doctor may want to check your blood for other reasons.

Are these drugs addictive?

These drugs are not addictive. There is no evidence of withdrawal symptoms.

I have heard the treatment is expensive. Will we have to pay for this treatment?

No, these drugs are now available on the NHS.

Summary of NICE guidance on anticholinesterases

- Anticholinesterase drugs may be prescribed for those with Alzheimer's disease with an MMSE score of more than 12 points.

- Diagnosis must be made in a specialist clinic.

- Assessments of cognitive functioning and activities of daily living should be made before starting drug treatment.

- Only specialists should initiate treatment.

- Only those likely to comply with drug treatment should be considered.

- Further assessments should be made 2–4 months after starting treatment. If MMSE scores indicated no deterioration or improvement and there is evidence of global or functional improvement then treatment should continue.

Those remaining on drug treatment should thereafter be assessed at 6-monthly intervals. Anticholinesterases should not normally be used in patients where MMSE scores fall below 12 points.

DEPOT MEDICATION

Task: Mr Hill is a 45-year-old gentleman who suffers from chronic schizophrenia. He has had multiple admissions in the past with recurrence of symptoms due to non-compliance with oral medications. Your consultant has proposed to start him on depot injections (Depixol). Explain to the patient about the drug and address his concerns.

Allay the patient's anxiety, as some patients are apprehensive of injections.

Note: The following questions and answers can be used for any of the depot medications, with some changes according to the particular drug.

What are depot medications?

Depots are injections, and they are a slow release form of antipsychotic. A 'depot' injection is a long-acting injection, usually given into a buttock or sometimes the thigh. If you are in hospital, a nurse will give the injection.

What are the advantages of having these injections as opposed to tablets?

The injection releases the drug over several weeks, so you will not have to remember to take tablets at regular times each day. Depot injections are neither more nor less effective than tablets or capsules. You only have to have the injection once a week, or even once a month. As you will have an appointment to go to your doctor or nurse to have the injection, you can remember easily when you have to have the injection.

If you missed your injection, your doctor or nurse would remind you. Above all, it may help you with your unpleasant experiences such as hearing voices, and you may be symptom-free when you are having the injection.

Who will give the injection and where will I have my injection?

You can usually decide yourself where to have the injections. The possible choices are:

1. At your local doctor's surgery

2. At a community mental health centre

3. At a special outpatient clinic

4. At your home, when a nurse visits you.

What happens when the nurse gives the depot medication?

You will go into a private, comfortable room. Usually there will be no one except yourself and a nurse. Initially you will be given a small amount of the medicine called a test dose to see if it has any bad effects on you, and to make sure the drug suits you. Then, if there are no problems, five to ten days later you will be given your first full dose injection, which will then be repeated every one to four weeks. These injections are usually given into the buttock, although some may be given into the thigh.

How do they work?

To put it briefly, these are made up of chemicals that help to balance out the chemicals in the brain. There is a naturally occurring chemical in the brain called dopamine. Dopamine is the chemical messenger mainly involved with thinking, emotions, behaviour, and perception. In some illnesses, dopamine may be overactive and upset the normal balance of chemicals. Excess dopamine helps to produce some of the symptoms of the illness. The main effect of these drugs is to block some dopamine receptors in the brain, reducing the effect of having too much dopamine, and correcting the imbalance. This reduces the symptoms caused by having too much dopamine.

How do they help?

Drugs help to alleviate the most disturbing symptoms of the illness. Medication works in two ways:

1. It reduces the symptoms of an attack of the illness.
2. Once the symptoms have improved it helps prevent further attacks or the symptoms getting worse.

Why do I need a test dose?

Depots are long-acting. Any adverse effects that result from injection are likely to be long-lived. Thus a small test dose is essential to help avoid severe, prolonged adverse effects.

If the medicine is OK for you, then you will start having regular injection. After each injection, the medicine will stay in your body for a few weeks.

Are there any side effects?

Like any other medication, these injections can also give you some difficulties. You may get some pain when the needle goes into your skin, especially when you have the injection. Other side effects are:

Common side effect	What happens
Drowsiness	Feeling sleepy or sluggish
Hypotension	Low blood pressure, feeling dizzy
Constipation	You may have some difficulty in passing motion or stools
Dry mouth	Not enough saliva or spit
Blurred vision	Things look fuzzy and you cannot focus properly
Weight gain	Eating more and putting on weight
Restlessness	Being on edge. You may feel restless
Movement disorders	Having shaky hands and feeling shaky

What should I do if I get any of these side effects?

Tell your doctor, your nurse or your key worker. They will want to help you with any problem with your medicine.

Can anything help with these side effects?

Yes. Often, having smaller amounts of the injection may help. Sometimes giving other tablets to counteract the side effects can also help.

How often do I have to have these injections?

We will administer at the longest possible licensed interval roughly between once a week and once a month.

How long will they take to work?

Some of the effects of these drugs appear soon after taking them, for example, the drowsiness. The most important action, to help the symptoms of your illness, may take weeks, or even months of regular medication to become fully effective. Similarly, if your dose or treatment is changed, it may take an equally long period of time before you notice the effects of such a change.

For how long will I need to keep taking them?

It is very difficult to say, as people's responses are different. You will probably need to continue your treatment for a long time, possibly several years after your symptoms have disappeared, to make sure you have fully recovered from your illness. Long-term treatment should be reviewed at regular intervals, for example, every three to six months, or even sooner if there are problems.

Are they addictive?

These drugs are not really addictive. If you have taken them for a long time, you may experience some mild effects if you stop taking them suddenly. The main problem would be your symptoms returning.

Can I stop taking them suddenly?

It is unwise to stop taking them suddenly, even if you feel better. Your symptoms can return if treatment is stopped too early. When the time comes, we will usually withdraw the drug by a gradual reduction in the dose taken over a period of several weeks.

Will they make me drowsy?

These drugs may make you feel drowsy or sleepy. You should not drive or operate machinery until you know how they affect you. You should take extra care, as they may affect your reaction times or reflexes. However, they are not sleeping tablets, although if you take them at night they may help you to sleep.

Will they cause weight gain?

Weight gain with these drugs is quite possible. In the people who gain weight, most is gained during the first 6–12 months of treatment. It then tends to level out. It is not possible to say what the effect on your own weight may be because each person will be affected differently. If you do start to put on weight or have other problems, you should tell your doctor. He/she may be able to adjust your drug or the dose of your drug to reduce this effect. Your doctor can also arrange for you to see a dietician for advice. If you do gain weight, it is possible to lose it while you are still taking this medication, with expert advice about diet.

Will it affect my sex life?

Drugs can affect desire (libido), arousal (erection), and orgasmic ability. These drugs are not thought to have a significant effect on any of these stages, but problems have been reported occasionally with these drugs. If this happens, however, you should discuss it with your doctor, as a change in dose or drug may help to minimise the problem.

Can I drink alcohol while I am taking these drugs?

If you drink alcohol while taking these drugs it may make you feel sleepier. This is particularly important if you need to drive or operate machinery, and you must seek advice on this.

Are there any foods or drinks that I should avoid?

You should have no problems with any food or drink other than alcohol.

Will they affect my other medication?

You should have no problems if you take other medications, although a few problems can occur. Sedative drugs might make you feel sleepier. This does not necessarily mean the drugs cannot be used together, just that you may need to follow your doctor's instructions very carefully. You should tell your doctor before starting or stopping these, or any other drugs. Make sure your doctor knows about all the medicines you are taking.

If I am taking a contraceptive pill, will this be affected?

It is not thought that 'the pill' is affected by any of these drugs.

Will I need a blood test?

Not usually.

Can I drive while I take them?

These drugs can affect your driving, e.g. you may feel drowsy. Until this wears off or you know how your drug affects you, do not drive or operate machinery. You should take extra care, as they may affect your reaction times or reflexes, even though you feel well.

It is an offence to drive, attempt to drive, or to be in charge of a vehicle when unfit through drugs. It is advisable to let your insurance company know if you are taking these drugs. If you do not and you have an accident, it could affect your insurance cover.

What will happen if I stop taking my injection?

If an individual stops taking his injection against the advice of their doctor then the chances of their having another attack are more than doubled. It is, therefore, very important that an individual keeps having their injection even when they feel completely well.

Note: When you explain about any medication (antipsychotics, antidepressants, mood stabilisers) make sure that you remember to cover the following important points which can gain you a global pass!

- Take the medication as directed by the doctor.

- If you are not sure about anything in regard to drugs, such as how many to take or if you have any problems taking your medication, then always ask the pharmacist or doctor.

- Never stop taking your medication without telling your doctor as this can lead to relapse of your illness.

- State the common, less common and then the serious side effects. State that many side effects will wear off after 2 weeks as your body adjusts to the drugs.

- Some drugs have serious side effects (e.g. lithium, clozapine). Explain these. State that: You must call (doctor, pharmacist or NHS) for help immediately if you think you are suffering any of these side effects.

- Explain if there are special precautions such as blood tests or dietary restrictions associated with the drugs.

- Do not drink alcohol while you are taking medication.

- Do not drive at least for two weeks after starting any medication or for two weeks after an increase in the dose.

ELICITING ALCOHOL HISTORY

Task: Mr Wells, a 43-year-old painter was admitted to the medical ward with acute gastritis. Routine blood tests showed increased GGT and MCV. He gave a history of drinking alcohol almost every day. The physicians have requested for an assessment. Elicit an alcohol history.

Explore the following:

1. Current usage

2. Longitudinal history

3. Edwards and Gross criteria

4. CAGE questionnaire

5. Risk factors

6. Complications

7. Insight and motivation

8. Rule out mood and psychotic symptoms

9. Any illicit drug abuse.

Note: In the next 11 chapters, it is almost impossible to cover all the questions in 7 minutes, but it is a good idea to ask at least three or four questions in each subheading to cover the important aspects and obtain a global pass!

Suggested approach

Step 1: Greet and introduce yourself
Step 2: Purpose of visit should be explained
Step 3: Obtain permission before you proceed
Step 4: Build rapport and address the patient's main concerns
Step 5: Start with open questions and then proceed to closed questions.

Questions

A. Current usage in a typical day/week

1. Do you drink?

2. What do you usually drink?

3. How much would you drink on a typical day?

4. How often do you drink?

5. How many units of alcohol would you have in a week?

6. How much money do you spend a day/week for drinking alcohol?

B. Longitudinal history

1. When did it all start?

2. What was the first drink?

3. With whom did you have the first drink?

4. Was it out of your own will (or) peer pressure?

5. How did you progress to the current level?

   a. Started drinking occasionally (social drink)

   b. Regular weekend drinking

   c. Regular evening drinking

   d. Regular lunchtime drinking

   e. Early morning drinking (progressive)

6. Have you tried other things and can you name the significant ones?

C. CAGE questions

- Do you feel that you have to cut down on your drinking?

- Do people annoy by criticising your drinking?

- Do you feel guilty about your drinking?

- Do you have to drink first thing in the morning to steady your nerves?

D. Edwards and Gross criteria for dependence syndrome

Compulsion

1. Do you sometimes crave for a drink? (or)

2. Do you have a compulsive urge to drink?

3. Do you find it hard to stop drinking once you start?

Tolerance

- Do you have to increase the intake of alcohol to get the same effect (or) the same amount has given you less effect than earlier? (or)

- Nowadays, do you need more alcohol to get drunk than you needed before?
- How much can you drink without feeling drunk?

Withdrawal symptoms

a. What happens if you miss your drink? (or)

b. What would happen if you go without a drink for a day or two? (or)

c. If you don't drink for a day (or) two, do you experience any withdrawal symptoms such as sweating, shaking, feeling sick and pounding in your heart?

Relief drinking

- Do you need a drink first thing in the morning to steady your nerves?
- Do you have to gulp the first few drinks of the day?

Stereotyped pattern

- Do you always drink in the same pub?
- Do you always drink with the same company?

Treatment and rapid re-instatement

a. Ask about details of treatment and details of any period of abstinence? (or) binge drinking.

b. Any detoxification programme? Was it completed or not?

c. If not, what are the reasons for the failure?

d. What helped you keep off drinks?

e. What made you start drinking again?

Primacy

1. How often do you miss family and social commitments because of drinking? (or)

2. Have you been giving primary importance to alcohol and have you been neglecting other alternative pleasures (or) interests? (or)

3. Does he/she drink despite knowing the ill-effects of alcohol?

E. Risk factors for alcohol abuse

Ask about:

- Occupation
- Psychiatric history

- Family history of alcoholism
- Premorbid personality

F. Ask about complications

Physical or mental health problems

- Accidents
- Memory problems
- Blackouts, falls, fits
- Loss of appetite, weight loss
- Anxiety, depression
- Head injury
- Suicidal ideation/behaviour.

Social problems

- Relationship difficulties with the partner, children, family members and friends
- Row or arguments with friends or mates
- Problems at working place – missing work, late, Monday absences
- Financial problems
- Legal problems – drink driving, drunk and disorderly behaviour, fights while drunk.

G. Insight and motivation

Do you feel you have a problem with alcohol?

Motivation

1. What would you like to do?
2. Have you ever thought of giving it up completely?
3. What do you think will happen if you give up completely?

H. Explore mood and psychotic symptoms

1. Rule out illicit drug abuse.

ELICITING PTSD HISTORY

Task: You have been asked to see Mr Young, a middle-aged business manager. The patient initially saw his GP because of difficulty in coping with the job. The patient met with an accident 6 months ago. Take a history to establish the features characteristic of the diagnosis and the extent of the problem.

Explore the following:

1. Details of the traumatic incident itself

2. Hyperarousal, intrusions and avoidance – core features of post-traumatic stress disorder (PTSD)

3. Assess the mode of onset of symptoms, duration, progress, severity and frequency of current symptoms

4. Impairment in social functioning

5. Rule out co-morbidity.

Suggested approach

Step 1: Greet and introduce yourself
Step 2: Purpose of visit should be explained
Step 3: Obtain permission before you proceed
Step 4: Build rapport and address the patient's main concerns
Step 5: Start with open questions and then proceed to closed questions.

• **Listen to the patient. Pick up clues from what the patient says to you.**

A. Traumatic incident

Explore the details of the accident, in particular the perceived severity and establish the level of distress and fear at the time of the event.

• Could you describe the accident please? (Here approach the patient empathetically as it is difficult to talk about traumatic incidents, and acknowledge the patients distress.)

• Find out about when it happened, how (terrifying) it was, any injuries, any head injury, loss of consciousness etc.

• Inquire about any blame, litigation, court cases and their outcome.

• Do you have any difficulties remembering parts of the accident?

B. Core features of PTSD

Intrusions

- How often do you think about the accident?
- Do you sometimes feel as if the accident is happening again?
- Do you get flashbacks?
- Have you revisited the scene?
- Do you get any distressing dreams/nightmares of the event?
- What would happen if you hear about an accident?

Avoidance

- How hard is it for you to talk about the accident?
- Do you deliberately try to avoid thinking about accidents?
- Do you make any effort to avoid the thoughts or conversations associated with the trauma? How would you do that?
- Do you make any effort to avoid activities, places or people that arouse recollection of the trauma?
- Have you been to the place where the accident happened?

Emotional detachment and numbness

- Have there been any changes in your feelings generally? (emotional detachment).
- How do you see the future?

Hyper arousal

- Have you had the feeling that you are always on the edge?
- Do you tend to worry a lot about things going wrong? (feeling anxious)
- Do you startle easily? (startled response)
- Tell me about your sleep please. (explore for sleep disturbance)
- Are you sometimes afraid to go to sleep?
- How has your concentration been recently?
- How has your memory been lately?
- Tell me about your temper please. (irritability)

C. Assess the mode of onset of symptoms, duration, progress, severity and frequency of current symptoms

Ask briefly about:

a. The mode of onset of symptoms

b. Duration and progress

c. Severity and frequency of symptoms

D. Distress and impairment of social functioning

- How do you feel in yourself generally?
- How has all this been affecting you?
- How do you spend your time these days?
- Enquire about effect on family, social life and work

Explore premorbid personality, past history

- Before all this happened, what sort of a person were you?
- How did you cope with stress?
- Have you had any mental health problems before the accident?

E. Explore co-morbidity

a. Mood symptoms, especially depression

b. Other anxiety symptoms

c. Current coping mechanisms including drugs and alcohol

Note: It is almost impossible to cover all the questions in 7 minutes, but it is a good idea to ask at least three or four questions in each subheading to cover the important aspects and obtain a global pass!

ELICITING EATING DISORDER HISTORY

Task: You are asked to see Ms Brown, a 21-year-old bank clerk who has insulin dependent diabetes mellitus. The GP was concerned about her diabetic control and the patient admitted to omitting her insulin to lose weight. You are asked to elicit an eating disorder history, rule out depression (no need to ask questions about IDDM).

Explore the following:

1. Psychological issues

2. Eating issues

3. Physical issues

4. Family dynamics and current stressors

5. Rule out co-morbidity.

Suggested approach

Step 1: Greet and introduce yourself
Step 2: Purpose of visit should be explained
Step 3: Obtain permission before you proceed
Step 4: Build rapport and address the patient's main concerns
Step 5: Start with open questions and then proceed to closed questions.

- **Listen to the patient. Pick up clues from what the patient says to you.**

A. Psychological issues

- What do you feel about your body and body weight?

- What is your ideal weight?

- Why is the weight ideal for you?

- Do you feel fat?/do you feel ugly?

- Does anyone comment on your being fat now?

- Do you dislike your body? If so, in what way?

- How do you feel when you see your image in a mirror?

- Do you feel that you have a distorted body image? If so, in what way?

- Do you 'fear loss of control? What do you mean by that?

- What do you feel would happen if you did not control your weight (or) eating?

B. Eating issues

- What is a typical day's eating?
- Is there a pattern? Does it vary?
- Do you avoid any particular foods? And if so, why?
- Do you restrict fluids?
- To what degree is the patient attempting restraint?

Binge eating

- Do you ever binge eat? (i.e. eat, during a short space of time, quantities of food that are definitely larger than most people would eat during a similar time and in similar circumstances).
- When did you first start binge eating?
- How often do you binge eat?
- Why do you binge eat?
- Is binge eating a problem for you?
- Tell me about a typical binge? Obtain information about type of foods eaten, the pace of eating, quantity of food, duration of the binge, vomiting or purging after the binge.
- How do you feel just before you binge?
- Can you identify any particular cause (e.g. feelings, stressors, social situations, etc.) that may trigger the binge?
- How do you feel while you are binge eating?
- How do you feel after a binge?

Vomiting

- Do you make yourself vomit? If so how?
- How often do you do this?
- Can you tell me why you make yourself vomit?
- Can you tell me what you do to make yourself vomit?

Laxatives, diuretics, emetics, appetite suppressants

- Do you take laxatives, diuretics, emetics, appetite suppressants?
- What kind?
- How many?
- How often?

- For what reason do you use it?
- Do you fast for a day or more?

Exercise

- Do you exercise?
- Is this to burn off calories?
- Do you use exercise as a means of controlling your weight?
- Do you find exercise useful for this purpose?
- How often do you exercise?
- How long each day/week do you spend exercising?
- What kind of exercise do you do?
- How do you feel before exercising? How do you feel after exercising?

C. Physical symptoms

- Weight loss/current weight
- Current height
- Menstrual changes – Are you menstruating regularly? Is it normal flow? Amount?
- Changes in libido – Loss of sexual interest and potency?
- Symptoms of anaemia: weakness, lethargy
- Constipation
- Muscle cramps.

D. Explore:

a. Family background

b. Current relationships

c. Other stresses

d. Your work

e. Social activities and life in general.

E. Do not forget to rule out depression and other neurotic symptoms

You can use the same questions in the chapter on depression and anxiety.

Note: It is almost impossible to cover all the questions in 7 minutes, but it is a good idea to ask at least three or four questions in each subheading to cover the important aspects and obtain a global pass!

ELICITING SYMPTOMS OF DEPRESSION

Task: Mr Jones presented to the A&E with low mood and sleep disturbance. Do a diagnostic assessment and elicit the symptoms of depression.

- Greet and introduce yourself

- Purpose of visit should be explained

- Obtain permission before you proceed

- Build rapport and address the patient's main concerns

- Start with open questions and then proceed to closed questions

- **Listen to the patient. Pick up clues from what the patient says to you**

Questions

A. Eliciting depressed mood and cognitive symptoms

- How are you feeling in yourself?

- Have you cried at all?

- If I were to ask you to rate your mood, on a scale of '0' to '10', where '0' is the rock bottom of how you feel and '10' is the best of your spirits, where would you place your mood over the last couple of weeks?

- Have you lost enjoyment in things you used to enjoy?

- How have you been in your energy levels these days?

- Have you been feeling drained of energy lately?

- How has your concentration been lately?

- How has been your memory recently?

B. Eliciting biological symptoms

- How has your sleep been recently?

- Have you had any trouble getting to sleep?

- Do you wake early in the morning?

- Is your depression worse at any particular time of day?

- What has your appetite been like recently?

- Have you lost any weight lately?

- Has there been any change in your interest in sex?

C. Eliciting suicidal intent and negative thoughts

- Have you felt that life wasn't worth living?
- Have you ever felt like ending it all?
- Did you actually try?
- How do you feel about it now?
- Would you do anything to harm yourself or hurt yourself?
- How confident do you feel in yourself?
- How do you describe your self-esteem to be?
- How do you see the future?
- Do you feel inferior to others (or) even worthless?
- Do you feel hopeless about yourself?
- Do you feel helpless?

D. Eliciting guilt feelings

- Do you feel that you've done something wrong?
- Do you feel guilty about things?
- Do you tend to blame yourself at all?
- Do you tend to blame anyone else for your problems?
- Do you have any regrets?
- Do you feel that you've committed a crime, (or) sinned greatly (or) deserve punishment?

E. Duration, course, effects, coping

- How long have you been feeling like this?
- What do you think might have caused this?
- How is it affecting your life?
- How do you manage to cope?
- Do you get any help?

F. Rule out co-morbidity

1. Contributing factors to illness and stressors
2. Anxiety
3. Psychosis

4. Mania/hypomania

5. Coping strategies like alcohol and illicit drug use.

Note: It is almost impossible to cover all the questions in 7 minutes, but it is a good idea to ask at least three or four questions in each subheading to cover the important aspects and obtain a global pass!

ELICITING HALLUCINATIONS

Task: Mr Smith presented himself to the A&E in a confused state complaining of hearing voices. You are asked to assess him and elicit different types of hallucinations.

- Greet and introduce yourself

- Purpose of visit should be explained

- Obtain permission before you proceed

- Build rapport and address the patient's main concerns

- Start with open questions and then proceed to closed questions

- **Listen to the patient. Pick up clues from what the patient says to you**

Auditory hallucinations

I understand that recently you have been hearing voices when there is no one around you and nothing else to explain it. Can you tell me more about it?
 (OR)
I should like to ask you a routine question, which we ask of everybody. Do you ever seem to hear voices (or) noises when there is no one about and nothing else to explain it?
 If the patient says 'yes' explore more about it.

Elementary hallucinations

- Do you hear noises like tapping or music?

- What is it like?

- Does it sound like muttering or whispering?

- Can you make out the words?

- Do you hear your name being called?

Second person auditory hallucinations

- Do they speak directly to you?

- Do they give orders?

- Do you obey?

- Can you carry on a two-way conversation with the voices?

- Who is it you are talking to?

- What is the explanation?
- Do you know anyone else who has this kind of experience?

Third person hallucinations

- Do you hear several voices talking about you?
- Do they refer to you as 'he' or 'she' like a 3rd person?
- What do they say?
- Do they seem to comment on what you are thinking, reading or doing?
- Do you hear voices like a running commentary instructing you to do things?
- Can you recognise those voices?
- If you recognise them, then whose voices are they?

Confirm whether they are true hallucinations

- Where do these voices come from?
- Do you hear them in your mind or in your ears?
- Do you hear them as clearly as you hear me?
- Can you start or stop them?
- Do you feel that they are real or do you feel that they are just voices?

Hypnagogic/hypnapompic hallucination

- Does your sleep get disturbed by these voices?
- Do you hear them more at any particular time of the day?

Visual hallucination

- Have you seen things (or) had visions that other people can't see?
- With your eyes (or) in your mind?
- Were you half asleep at that time?
- What did you see?
- Has it occurred when you are fully awake?
- Did you realise that you were seeing things?
- How do you explain it?

Olfactory hallucination

- Is there anything unusual about the way things feel or taste or smell?
- Do you sometimes notice strange smells that other people don't notice?

Gustatory hallucination

- Have you noticed that food or drink seems to have an unusual taste recently?

Tactile hallucination

- Do you ever feel that someone is touching you, but when you look there is nobody there?

Functional hallucination

- Do voices occur only upon a background of stimulus in the same modality?

Reflex hallucination

- Do voices occur in response to a stimulus in a different modality?

Ask about alcohol and illicit drug abuse.

Duration, course, effects, coping

- How long have you been feeling like this?
- What do you think might have caused this?
- How is it affecting your life?
- How do you manage to cope?
- Do you get any help?

Rule out co-morbidity

1. Contributing factors to illness and stressors
2. Anxiety
3. Depression

4. Mania/hypomania

5. Coping strategies like alcohol and illicit drug use.

Note: It is almost impossible to cover all the questions in 7 minutes, but it is a good idea to ask at least three or four questions in each subheading to cover the important aspects and obtain a global pass!

ELICITING FIRST RANK SYMPTOMS

Task: Mr Brown was referred by his GP complaining of hearing voices and being controlled by some evil forces. Elicit the first rank symptoms.

Schneider's first rank symptoms are:

1. Hearing thoughts spoken aloud
2. Third person auditory hallucinations
3. Running commentary hallucinations
4. Thought withdrawal
5. Thought insertion
6. Thought broadcasting
7. Made volition
8. Made feelings
9. Made impulses
10. Somatic passivity
11. Delusional perception.

Suggested approach

- Greet and introduce yourself
- Purpose of visit should be explained
- Obtain permission before you proceed
- Build rapport and address the patient's main concerns
- Start with open questions and then proceed to closed questions
- **Listen to the patient. Pick up clues from what the patient says to you**

I gather that you had been through a lot of stress and strain recently. When under stress sometimes people have certain unusual experiences. Have you had any such experiences? By unusual experience, I mean for example, hearing noises or voices when there is no one around.

If the patient says, 'yes' explore more about the voices. Can you tell me more about the voices?

Third person auditory hallucinations

- Do the voices speak among themselves?
- Do you hear several voices talking about you?
- Do they refer to you as 'he' (or) 'she' as a 3rd person?
- What do they say?

Running commentary hallucinations

1. Do they seem to comment on what you are thinking, reading or doing?

(Or)

2. Do you hear voices like a running commentary instructing you to do things?

Hearing thoughts spoken aloud

- Can you hear what you are thinking?
- Do the voices repeat your thoughts?
- Do you ever seem to hear your own thoughts echoed or repeated?
- What is it like?
- How do you explain it?
- Where does it come from?

Thought alienation phenomenon (open question)

- Are you able to think clearly?
- Is there any interference with your thoughts?

Thought broadcasting

- Do you feel that your thoughts are private (or) are they accessible to others in any way?
- Are your thoughts broadcast, so that other people know what you are thinking?

(Or)

- Can anyone read your thoughts?
- How do you know?
- How do you explain it?

Thought insertion

- Are thoughts put into your head which you know are not your own?
- How do you know they are not your own?
- Where do they come from?

Thought withdrawal

- Do your thoughts ever seem to be taken from your head, as though some external person (or) forces were removing them?

(Or)

- Could someone take your thoughts out of your head?
- Would that leave your mind empty or blank?
- Can you give an example?
- How do you explain it?

Passivity of feelings or actions

- When under stress sometimes people have certain unusual experiences. Have you had any such experiences?
- Are you always in control of what you feel and do? (open question)

(Or)

- Is there something or someone trying to control you?
- Do you feel under the control of some force or power other than yourself as though you are a robot or a zombie without a will of your own?
- Does this force make your movements for you without you willing it?
- Does this force or power force its feelings on to you against your will?
- Does this force have any other influence on your body?

Somatic hallucinations

1. Some people have funny sensations on the body, for example, insects crawling or electricity passing or muscles being stretched or squeezed.
2. Have you had any such experiences?
3. How do you explain it?

Delusional perception

1. Do you think that things happening around you have a special meaning to you?
2. Can you explain it please?

Effects, coping (probe in detail)

- What do you think is causing these experiences?
- Who do you think is causing them?
- Why do they do so? And how do they do that?
- How would you explain them?
- Could it be your imagination?
- How long have you had these experiences?
- How do they affect you?
- How do they make you feel?
- How would you cope with them?
- What do you intent to do about them?

Listen to the patient. Pick up clues from what the patient says to you.

Note: It is almost impossible to cover all the questions in 7 minutes, but it is a good idea to ask at least three or four questions in each subheading to cover the important aspects and obtain a global pass!

ELICITING DELUSIONS AND OTHER EXPERIENCES

Task: You are seeing Mr Atkins, a 49-year-old postal worker brought to the A&E by the police. He presented to the police station earlier today stating that he could no longer hide from the police and he was 'giving himself up'. Explore the content of his beliefs and other experiences.

Suggested approach

- Greet and introduce yourself

- Purpose of visit should be explained

- Obtain permission before you proceed

- Build rapport and address the patient's main concerns

In this station, explore why he has come to the hospital, why he went to the police station today and said that he was 'giving himself up' and what has been worrying him/bothering him. Listen to the patient. Pick up clues from what the patient says to you.

Questions

Start with open questions and then proceed to closed questions given below.

Delusions of persecution

- How well have you been getting on with people?

- Do you ever feel uncomfortable as if people are watching you? (or) talking about you behind your back?

- Is anyone trying to harm, or interfere with you?

- Is anyone deliberately trying to poison you (or) to kill you? (or) make your life miserable?

- Is there any organisation like the Mafia behind it?

Delusions of reference

- Do people seem to drop hints about you or say things with a special meaning?

- Does everyone seem to gossip about you?

- Do you see any reference to yourself on TV or in the newspapers?
- Do things seem to be specially arranged?

Delusions of control or passivity

- Is there anyone trying to control you?
- Do they force you to think, say or do things?
- Do they change the way you feel in yourself?
- Do you feel that you are under the control of a person or force other than yourself?
- Do you feel as if you're a robot or zombie with no will of your own?

Delusions of grandiosity

- How do you see yourself compared to others?
- Do you have any special powers or abilities?
- Are you specially chosen in any way?
- Is there a special mission to your life?
- Are you a prominent person (or) related to someone prominent like Royalty?
- Are you very rich (or) famous?
- What about special plans?

Delusions of guilt

- Do you feel you have done something wrong?
- Do you have any regrets?
- Do you feel guilty?
- Do you feel you deserve punishment?

Religious delusions

- Are you especially close to God or Christ?
- Can God communicate with you?

Nihilistic delusions

- Do you feel something terrible has happened or will happen to you?
- How do you see the future?

- Do you feel that you have died?

- Has part of your body died or been removed?

- Inquire about being doomed, being a pauper, intestines being blocked etc.

Hypochondriacal delusions

1. How is your health?

2. Are you concerned that you might have a serious illness?

Delusions of jealousy

1. Can you tell me about your relationship?

2. Do you feel that your partner reciprocates your loyalty?

Delusional mood

1. Do you ever get the feeling that something odd is going on that you can't explain? (Do familiar surroundings seem strange?)

2. Is there something odd about the way things look, or sound, or smell or taste?

Delusional perception

- Do you think that things happening around you have a special meaning to you?

(Or)

- Has a sudden explanation occurred out of the blue to you?

Thought withdrawal, insertion and broadcasting

- Are you able to think clearly?

- Is there any interference with your thoughts?

- Do you feel that your thoughts are private (or) are they accessible to others in any way?

- Are your thoughts broadcast, so that other people know what you are thinking?

- Can anyone read your thoughts?

- Are thoughts put into your head which you know are not your own?

- Could someone take your thoughts out of your head and would that leave your mind empty or blank?

If the patient says 'yes' to any of the delusions, then pick up the clues from what the patient says to you. Probe further, elaborate and clarify. Assess the degree of conviction, explanation, effects and coping. Also assess their onset (primary/secondary) and their fixity (partial/complete).

Conviction, explanation, effects, coping

Do not be satisfied with a 'Yes' answer. Probe, elaborate and clarify.

- What do you think is causing these experiences?
- Who do you think is causing them?
- Why do they do so? And how do they do that?
- How would you explain them?
- Could it be your imagination?
- Ask how he copes, what he has done and what he intends to do about them.

Always check whether the delusion is:

Partial or full

- Even when you seemed to be most convinced, do you really feel in the back of your mind that it might well not be true, that it might be your imagination?

Primary or secondary

- How did it come into your mind that this was the explanation?
- Did it happen suddenly or out of the blue?
- How did it begin?

Listen to the patient. Pick up clues from what the patient says to you.

Note: It is almost impossible to cover all the questions in 7 minutes, but it is a good idea to ask at least three or four questions in each subheading to cover the important aspects and obtain a global pass!

ELICITING ANXIETY SYMPTOMS

Task: Mrs Brown is a 45-year-old lady who has been referred to you for feeling anxious, edgy all the time and fears of 'going crazy'. Elicit a detailed history.

Suggested approach

- Greet and introduce yourself
- Purpose of visit should be explained
- Obtain permission before you proceed.
- Build rapport and address the patient's main concerns

In this station, explore why she has come to the hospital, why she has been feeling anxious, edgy and what has been worrying her/bothering her. Listen to the patient. Pick up clues from what the patient says to you.

Questions

Start with open questions and then proceed to closed questions given below.

Eliciting anxiety symptoms

- Have there been times when you have been very anxious (or) frightened?
- Have you had the feeling that something terrible might happen?
- Have you had the feeling that you are always on the edge?
- Do you worry a lot about simple things?
- Tell me what made you feel so anxious?
- Tell me about your anxiety symptoms?
- How long you've been feeling so anxious?
- How does it interfere with your life and activities?

Eliciting panic attacks

- Have you had times when you felt shaky, your heart pounded, you felt sweaty and you simply had to do something about it?
- Were you getting butterflies in stomach, jelly legs, palpitations, shaky, trembling of hands and sweating?

- What was it like?
- What was happening at the time?
- How often do you get these attacks?

Agoraphobia

- Do you tend to get anxious when going into a crowded place, public spaces, travelling away from home (or) travelling alone?
- Do you tend to avoid any of these situations because you know that you'll get anxious?
- How much does it affect your life?

Social phobia

- Do you tend to get anxious when meeting people (e.g.) going into a crowded room and making conversation?
- What about speaking to audience?
- What about eating (or) drinking in front of other people?

Special phobias

- Do you have any special fears like some people are scared of cats or spiders or birds?

Explore in detail about the symptom history, mode of onset, duration, progression of symptoms. Rule out co-morbidity:

a. Depression

b. Obsessional symptoms

c. Coping mechanisms.

Listen to the patient. Pick up clues from what the patient says to you.

Note: It is almost impossible to cover all the questions in 7 minutes, but it is a good idea to ask at least three or four questions in each subheading to cover the important aspects and obtain a global pass!

ELICITING OBSESSIVE-COMPULSIVE SYMPTOMS

Task: Miss Smith is a 27-year-old woman who has come to your clinic following referral by her GP. She mentioned that she has certain problems with cleanliness and really wanted to speak to someone. Talk to her about her symptoms.

Suggested approach

- Greet and introduce yourself
- Purpose of visit should be explained
- Obtain permission before you proceed
- Build rapport and address the patient's main concerns
- Start with open questions and then proceed to closed questions
- **Listen to the patient. Pick up clues from what the patient says to you**

I gather that your doctor has referred you to my clinic today. Can you tell me briefly about what has been bothering you?

Questions

Then explore more with the following questions:

Obsessional symptoms

- Can you tell me something more about the thoughts you have been having?
- Do any unpleasant thoughts/ideas keep coming into your mind, even though you try hard not to have them?
- Where do they come from?
- Are these thoughts your own or are they put into your mind by some external force?
- How often do you have these thoughts?
- What do you do when you get these thoughts?
- Are they distressing and if so in what way?

- Is there anything you try to do to stop these thoughts?

- What happens when you try to stop them?

Compulsive symptoms

- Do you find that you have to keep on checking things that you know that you have already done?

- Like gas taps, doors, and switches?

- What happens when you try to stop them?

- Do you spend a lot of time on personal cleanliness, like washing over and over even though you know that you're clean?

- Does contamination with germs worry you?

- Do you have to touch (or) count things many times?

- Do you have any other rituals?

- Do you find it difficult to make decisions even for simple trivial things? (obsessional ruminations).

Explore in detail about the symptom history, mode of onset, duration, precipitating factors and associated problems. Ask about associated symptoms, such as:

- Depression

- Generalised anxiety

- Panic attacks

- Phobias

- Anankastic personality traits – Do you tend to do things/keep things in an organised way?

Listen to the patient. Pick up clues from what the patient says to you.

Note: It is almost impossible to cover all the questions in 7 minutes, but it is a good idea to ask at least three or four questions in each subheading to cover the important aspects and obtain a global pass!

MANIC/HYPOMANIC SYMPTOMS

Task: Mr Brown is a 25-year-old gentleman who was admitted to the ward with elated mood, hyperactivity and lots of unrealistic active plans for the future. Elicit more history from the patient.

Suggested approach

- Greet and introduce yourself
- Purpose of visit should be explained
- Obtain permission before you proceed
- Build rapport and address the patient's main concerns
- Start with open questions and then proceed to closed questions
- **Listen to the patient. Pick up clues from what the patient says to you**

Questions

Eliciting hypomanic/manic symptoms

- How are you feeling in yourself?
- Have you sometimes felt particularly cheerful and on top of the world, without any reason?
- Have you felt particularly full of energy lately (or) full of exciting ideas?
- Do you find yourself extremely active but not getting tired?
- Do you need less sleep than usual?
- Have you developed new interests lately?
- Have you felt especially healthy?
- Have you been buying interesting things recently?
- Do you feel that your thoughts are racing and you find difficulty in thinking?

Eliciting grandiose ideas and delusions

- How do you see yourself compared to others?
- Are you specially chosen in any way?
- Do you have any special powers or abilities quite out of the ordinary?

- Is there a special mission to your life?
- Are you a prominent person (or) related to someone prominent like the Royalty?
- Are you very rich (or) famous?
- What about special plans?

Explore in detail about the symptom history, mode of onset, duration, progress, precipitating factors and associated problems. Rule out co-morbidity such as:

- Depression
- Psychotic symptoms
- Coping mechanisms
- Drug and alcohol misuse.

Listen to the patient. Pick up clues from what the patient says to you.

Note: It is almost impossible to cover all the questions in 7 minutes, but it is a good idea to ask at least three or four questions in each subheading to cover the important aspects and obtain a global pass!

ELICITING ILLICIT DRUG HISTORY

Task: You are asked to assess this 27-year-old gentleman with history of using illicit substances such as heroin. Take detailed history about the usage of illicit substances.

The areas to be explored are:

1. Current usage

2. Longitudinal history

3. Any evidence of dependence

4. Complications

5. Treatment

6. Motivation

7. Alcohol use

8. Rule out psychotic, mood symptoms.

Suggested approach

- Greet and introduce yourself

- Purpose of visit should be explained

- Obtain permission before you proceed

- Start with open questions

Questions

Open questions

- Are there any tablets (or) medicines that you take apart from those you get from your doctor?

- Is there anything that you buy from the chemists (or) get from friends?

- Have you ever used any recreational drugs such as cannabis, cocaine/crack, amphetamines, speed, ecstasy, LSD (or) acid? (**Ask about individual drugs by naming them**).

- What about tablets to settle your nerves (or) help you sleep?

Current usage

- What drugs are you using now?
- What is the frequency of use?
- What is the amount of drug taken? (in appropriate measures such as ounces)
- What is the pattern of a typical drug using day (or) week?
- What is the route of use? (oral, smoked, snorted, injected)

If injected, the following questions are useful to ask:

    a. Are needles used?

    b. Where are they obtained from?

    c. Are needles shared?

    d. What sites are used for injection?

- What effect is the patient seeking when using the drug?
- Ask if more than one drug is used at a time.

Longitudinal history

- Ask about how long is the history of drug use, and how it has evolved.
- When did it start?
- What was the first drug taken?
- Was it by your own will (or) peer pressure?
- How did you progress to the current level?

Any evidence for dependence

Compulsion

- Do you sometimes crave for drugs?
- Do you have a compulsive urge to take drugs?

Tolerance

- Do you have to increase the amount of drugs that you take to get the same effect (or) same amount has given you less effect than earlier?

Withdrawal symptoms

- If you don't take drugs for a day (or) two, do you experience any withdrawal symptoms?

For example, if the patient takes heroin, ask about symptoms such as sweating, gooseflesh, running nose, watery eyes etc.

Complications

- Have you experienced any complication? (Ask about physical, mental and social complications?)
- What risky behaviour does the patient engage in?

Treatment

- What is the patient's past experience of treatment for a drug problem?
- Have there been any periods of abstinence and if so, what has helped the patient to achieve this?
- What triggers have brought on relapses?

Insight

- Do you feel you have a problem with drugs?

Motivation

- What would you like to do?
- Have you ever thought of giving it up completely?
- What do you think will happen if you give up completely?
- **Ask about alcohol history**
- **Rule out mood and psychotic symptoms**
- **Thank the patient and the examiner**

PREMORBID PERSONALITY

Task: Elicit the premorbid personality of this 45-year-old gentleman who has come to see you in your outpatient clinic.
   Ideally, collateral history is necessary to elicit premorbid personality.

Questions

Start with open questions:

- How would you describe yourself as a person before you were ill?

- How do other people describe you as a person?

Then ask closed questions about individual personality traits:

- How do you get on with people? (paranoid)

- Do you trust other people? (paranoid)

- Would you describe yourself as a 'loner'? (schizoid)

- Do you have many friends? (schizoid)

- Do you indulge in fantasies? Sexual and non-sexual fantasies, daydreaming?

- What's your temper like? (antisocial, emotionally unstable)

- Are you an impulsive person? (impulsive)

- Do you take responsibility for your actions? (antisocial, impulsive)

- Are you over-emotional (histrionic)

- How do you cope with life? (anxious, borderline)

- How do you cope with your emotions? (borderline, anxious)

- Do you maintain long-term relationships with people? (antisocial, borderline)

- Are you anxious (or) shy? (anxious/avoidant)

- Are you a worrier? (anxious, dependent)

- How do you respond to criticisms? (anxious/paranoid)

- How much do you depend on others? (dependent)

- Do you tend to keep things in an orderly way? (anankastic)

- Do you have unusually high standards at work/home? (anankastic)

Also ask about:

1. Predominant mood
    a. Optimistic/pessimistic
    b. Stable/prone to anxiety
    c. Cheerful/despondent
    d. Reaction to stressful life events
2. Interpersonal relationships
    a. Current friendships and relationships
    b. Previous relationship – ability to establish and maintain
    c. Family relationships
    d. Sociability – friends, work mates and superiors
3. Coping strategies
    a. How does the patient cope with problems?
    b. Do they tolerate stress?
    c. Does he have sufficient coping strategies?
4. Personal interests
    a. Hobbies, interests
    b. Use of leisure time
5. Beliefs – religious beliefs
6. Habits – food fads, alcohol, current (or) previous use of drugs (etc.)
- **Thank the patient and the examiner.**

EXPLAIN COGNITIVE BEHAVIOURAL THERAPY

Task: Mrs Doherty, a 30-year-old woman suffers from recurrent depressive disorder and shows only partial response to two different antidepressant drugs. You are planning to refer her for CBT. The patient wants to know more about CBT.

- Greet and introduce yourself

- Purpose of visit should be explained

- Obtain permission before you proceed

- First explain to the patient about your plan to refer her to CBT

What does CBT stand for?

CBT stands for cognitive behavioural therapy.

What is cognitive therapy?

There are two main types of treatments for depression. One is the physical treatments such as medication or ECT, and the other is the psychological or talking treatments. CBT is one of the most commonly used psychological treatments.

Can you tell me more about it please?

Cognitive therapy is a way of helping people to cope with stress and emotional problems. The idea behind it is quite simple – the way we think about things affects how we feel emotionally.

When people are depressed, they often have negative thoughts about themselves, their future and the world in general. These thoughts come automatically into their minds. These negative thoughts or 'cognitions', undermine their self-confidence, and make them feel even more depressed leading to unhelpful behaviours. The therapist will work with you to identify the thinking and behavioural patterns that contribute to how you feel, and help you to make changes.

Is it the same as counselling?

CBT is a lot different from counselling. They are both talking treatments, although CBT is much more structured. Counselling is a way of talking through your problems with a counsellor, who can help by listening to your problems. A counsellor may also help you to get a more helpful perspective on problems in your daily life.

How does it work?

Cognitive therapy is a way of talking about the connections between how we think, how we feel and how we behave. It particularly concentrates on ideas that are unrealistic. These often undermine our self-confidence and make us feel depressed or anxious. Looking at these negative thoughts and challenging these negative thoughts can help us work out different ways of thinking and behaving that in turn will help us cope better.

Will I have to lie on a couch and talk about childhood?

Not really. CBT looks at 'here and now' issues rather than things from the past. It helps people to learn new methods of coping and solving problems, which they can use for the rest of their lives.

What is the duration of this therapy?

CBT usually lasts for 8 to 12 weeks. Usually there will be one session a week, each lasting about 50 minutes.

Who will be seeing me?

Someone with special training and experience in CBT such as a psychologist, a nurse therapist, a psychiatric social worker or a psychiatrist will be seeing you.

What does a course of therapy involve?

In the first few sessions, the client and the therapist decide which problems seem to be the most important. Clients take an active part and carry out 'homework' tasks between sessions. They will often be asked to keep a diary of their thoughts, feelings and behaviours in the situations that they find particularly stressful. They then discuss these in detail in the sessions with the therapist, asking themselves whether or not their ways of thinking are realistic. They can then learn to change these ways of thinking to use more helpful ones. Cognitive therapy also helps us to look at our 'rules for living'.

Can you explain to me about 'rules for living'?

These are strong beliefs about how we should live our lives which we develop while we are growing up. They are based both on what we learn from other people and on our own experiences. For example, someone may grow up with the belief that 'I cannot be happy unless I am successful in everything I do'. This belief is unrealistic – the reality of life is that we all fail sometimes. By demanding the impossible, this idea is likely to produce feelings of depression. Cognitive therapy can help us not only to be aware of the 'rules' we use but also to develop more helpful ones.

Whom can it help?

Research has shown that it is particularly helpful for people who suffer from anxiety or depression. It may also be used to treat panic attacks and eating disorders such as bulimia.

Cognitive therapy particularly suits people who want to be actively involved in dealing with their problems.

Can you have CBT when you are taking antidepressants?

Yes, you can. In fact, the scientific and research evidence is that CBT and anti-depressants enhance each other's effects.

Is it useful for anxiety-related problems?

More often depression and anxiety go hand in hand. CBT particularly suits people who want to be actively involved in dealing with their problems. We use CBT techniques to treat both depression and anxiety.

Can CBT prevent depression coming back?

Yes it can. CBT helps by changing your thinking and behaviour patterns and in fact, the last few sessions focus on relapse prevention. Hence, it is effective in reducing the chances of relapse.

But eventually it will be you sorting out your own problems with the help of the CBT therapist. This will need to happen over the long term. You may need to come in from time to time for check-up sessions. You can still continue taking your medications and you will still have access to supports like your GP.

What do I do in an emergency or crisis?

In an emergency or crisis, you will need to use your normal network of support. This could include family and friends in the first instance, but also other agencies – such as your GP or the crisis intervention team – depending on what you need at the time.

Can I stop if I feel it's not working?

It is always possible to leave therapy, though the pressure to remain may seem stressful at times. Talk about your difficulties with your therapist before you decide to stay or leave. Ultimately, if you want to stop, it is up to you.

■ Note: Worth mentioning about information leaflets and fact sheets at the end.

OBSESSIVE-COMPULSIVE DISORDER

Task: Mrs Wilkinson has been diagnosed as suffering from obsessive-compulsive disorder. She wants to know more about the illness and the treatments available. Address her concerns and allay her anxiety.

Suggested approach

- Greet and introduce yourself
- Purpose of visit should be explained
- Obtain permission before you proceed
- Address the patient's main concerns first

What is obsessive-compulsive disorder?

Obsessive-compulsive disorder (OCD) is based around obsessive (engrossing) thoughts, for example fear of contamination, as well as a compulsion (urge) to carry out physical rituals such as excessive washing. The ritual behaviour often helps to relieve the fear created by the obsessive thoughts.

People with OCD are usually aware that their obsessive thoughts are irrational, but nevertheless feel powerless to control them.

The compulsions, such as excessive hand washing, are time consuming and can interfere with all aspects of your life – your daily routine, work, and relationships with others, but if the compulsion is not performed, that too creates great anxiety.

How common is this condition?

OCD affects between one to two people in 100 and usually begins in late childhood or adolescence.

Some of the most common obsessions are:

- Worrying about contamination with dirt or germs
- Being overly concerned about symmetry or orderly arrangement of things
- Worrying about unusual sexual thoughts
- Aggressive impulses
- Doubting about things you know you shouldn't worry about.

Some of the most common compulsions are:

- Checking

- Washing
- Measuring
- Hoarding
- Counting
- Need to ask or confess.

Why are rituals performed?

Someone who has OCD typically has intrusive thoughts or images that generate anxiety, discomfort, or the urge to carry out rituals. When these rituals are carried out the level of anxiety or discomfort is usually reduced. Therefore, the performance of these rituals is strengthened and the rituals continue to occur.

For example, an individual may have the thought that his or her hands have touched something dirty or contaminated. This thought causes anxiety because the person may feel uncomfortable about the idea of being contaminated or of contaminating someone else. This anxiety or discomfort is relieved by washing the hands or other contaminated objects. It feels good for that person to rid himself or herself of such negative feelings, hence, it feels 'good' to wash.

What causes OCD?

There are several ideas about the causes of OCD:

1. One idea is that it is a 'learned' behaviour, in which the person comes to recognise the performance of rituals with relief from anxiety – thus reinforcing the behaviour.

2. Another idea says that OCD has a genetic cause – that is, it runs in families. It is known that 25% of people with OCD also have a close relative with the disorder.

3. Thirdly, there is an idea that OCD results from changes in the balance of chemicals in the brain. It has been known for some time that one of these chemicals, serotonin, is important in depression – depressed people have low levels of serotonin. And it is now also believed that low levels of serotonin are an important factor in people with OCD.

There is in fact a strong link between OCD and depression – two-thirds of people with OCD will be depressed at some point in their lives. One-third will have a major depression when they are first diagnosed as having OCD. It is therefore important to have any depression treated, in addition to OCD itself.

How is OCD treated?

OCD can be treated through relaxation techniques, psychological or talking treatment and drug treatment – or by a combination of all three.

Drug treatment

The antidepressant medications have been shown to be helpful in treating OCD. As with all medicines, you may find that your drug treatment has some side effects, but these may last only for a short period of time.

The most common side effects found with antidepressant medicines are nausea, headaches, dry mouth, blurred vision, dizziness and feeling sleepy. However it is important to remember that they are not addictive. They will not cause withdrawal symptoms when you stop taking them.

If you are concerned about side effects which are severe or last for a long time, go back and see your doctor. She/he may be able to change your medicine or the dosage.

How long should I take the medications?

If you are given drug treatment for OCD, you may have to stay on treatment for a long time. This is to make sure there's no chance of symptoms returning.

You may find it takes a few weeks for your drugs to start working – your doctor can tell you how soon you can expect to see results. Whatever medicine you're taking, it is important that you keep taking it until your doctor tells you to stop.

What are the psychological or talking treatments that are available?

Different forms of psychological treatments and the most commonly used treatments are:

1. Exposure and response prevention

2. Cognitive behavioural therapy.

Can you tell me more in detail about exposure and response prevention please?

The treatment strategy involves exposing the individual to stimuli that trigger anxiety or discomfort, and then having the individual voluntarily refrain from performing his or her ritual or compulsion.

To put it briefly, the first step is to help the individual plan a graded programme of exposure tasks that can be attempted in a systematic way.

For each ritual the individual will be required to list a range of situations that cause anxiety and which trigger the urge to perform that ritual.

The individual would then rate each of these situations according to the amount of anxiety or distress that would arise if he or she did not perform the particular ritual.

These are then arranged in order according to those that generate the *least* anxiety or discomfort to those that generate the most anxiety or discomfort. The first task in the list would be an activity that is mildly discomforting but not too difficult, while the last task in the list would be the most difficult task that the individual can imagine.

Let me explain the steps involved in exposure and response prevention

Step 1: Firstly, provide training for slow breathing exercises and relaxation. These exercises can be used prior to commencing each step of the graded exposure hierarchy to ensure that the individual is calm and relatively relaxed at the beginning of each graded exposure session.

Step 2: Identify a first small step towards overcoming the feared ritual.

Step 3: Practise this step until it no longer causes anxiety.

Step 4: Move on to a more difficult step and repeat the practice.

Step 5: Continue this process until the person can manage the last step towards overcoming the ritual.

It is worth mentioning the following points:

- This is a simple but highly effective technique

- It is used particularly in treatment of phobias and OCD

- The active participation of clients is necessary

- The situation can be real or imagined (a real-life situation will be more effective)

- It is usually done in graded steps

- It can be practised regularly with self-exposure tasks.

Cognitive behavioural therapy
See previous chapters for CBT explanation.

What will happen in the future?

It may seem difficult to believe right now, but with the right treatment it is possible for most people to overcome OCD. Progress may be slow, but complete recovery is possible. Remember to follow your doctor's advice; including taking any medicine you are given every day.

- **Note: It is worth mentioning at the end about information leaflets, fact sheets and other information available in books and on the Internet.**

AGORAPHOBIA – MANAGEMENT

Task: Mrs Brown is a 45-year-old woman who lives with her husband. She suffers from agoraphobia. She has come to see you to discuss the treatment options available. Address her concerns and allay her anxiety.

- Greet and introduce yourself

- Purpose of visit should be explained

- Obtain permission before you proceed

- Address the patient's main concerns first

Treatment options

What are the treatment options available for agoraphobia?

Agoraphobia is a common problem and it is definitely treatable. There are a number of different treatments available including education, psychological treatments and medication.

Education may sound simple, but you and your family need to know about the nature of the illness, what keeps it going and how to deal with it.

What are the medications available for treatment of agoraphobia?

There are two main types of medication, benzodiazepines and antidepressants. Benzodiazepines, for example (Valium) start working very quickly and can be useful in the short term but they are addictive, and you may become dependent on them. However, antidepressants would be a very good option.

Does that mean that I am depressed?

No, not at all. Even though they are called antidepressants, these drugs are useful to treat a variety of conditions like depression, anxiety, panic attacks and agoraphobias. They treat and modify the chemical imbalance in the brain that are common to all these disorders.

How do you go about it?

We start them at a low dose and increase gradually. They may take up to 8 weeks to start working. Once you feel better, you will have to continue the medication for about 6 months, if not longer. Then we have to taper it off gradually and stop. They are not addictive.

What about psychological treatments?

The psychological treatments are more structured and they are of two types:

1. Systematic desensitisation

The first one is **systematic desensitisation** also called **graded exposure with relaxation.** In this therapy, first we will teach you relaxation exercises to help you control your anxiety and panic. Then we make a list of hierarchy of situations that you find difficult to face. We order them from the least difficult to the most difficult.

Then you start by facing the easiest situation, whilst managing to relax. When you feel comfortable with that situation, you then go onto the next one. You will have to do this daily. You may find it easier to face situations if you move from the least difficult to the most difficult, e.g. like going out of the front door of your house, going out to your garden from your house, then going out to a nearby shop with a family member and then going out to a supermarket with a family member and so on. Practice the steps until it no longer causes anxiety. Move on to a more difficult step and repeat the practice.

The secret to success is *regular* and *gradual* progress.

Do new steps need to be practised more frequently and for longer periods of time before moving on to more difficult steps?
It is important that the individual masters the present step before moving on to a more difficult step. Some steps are more difficult than others, hence the individual may need to progress more slowly at times. Moving on without sufficient practice can lead to loss of confidence and motivation if the individual experiences a setback at the next step.

What happens if a setback occurs?
If a setback occurs it may be helpful for the individual to return to a previous step at which he or she feels more comfortable. It will also be helpful to encourage the individual to view the setback in a positive light.

How do you deal with more difficult steps?
In some cases, intermediate steps may need to be added to the more difficult steps so that the increase in difficulty is more manageable.

I can't come out of my house as I am worried that I might collapse. How can you help me in this situation?

We can understand your difficulties. In that case, we can arrange for the therapist to come to your house to help you.

What is the other treatment you mentioned?

The other form of psychological treatment is cognitive behavioural therapy that explores your thoughts when you are anticipating a fearful event and explores the factors that seems to maintain the problem (see CBT chapter for more information).

You mentioned my family members; what can they do?
Your family members and or your partner have an important role in the treatment. It would be very helpful if they also learn how the therapy works, so that they are able to support, motivate and help you to tackle problems that keep the illness going. They could support you and accompany you for the treatment sessions. So it will be very helpful if they can also be involved.

- **Note:** It is worth mentioning at the end about information leaflets, fact sheets and other information available in books and on the Internet.

PANIC DISORDER – HYPERVENTILATION

Task: Mr Williams is a 45-year-old gentleman who suffers from panic disorder. His father recently died of heart attack and there is a strong family history of ischaemic heart disease. He is therefore concerned that he might suffer from heart attacks. Address his concerns and explain to him about how hyperventilation can worsen panic attacks.

- Greet and introduce yourself
- Purpose of visit should be explained
- Obtain permission before you proceed
- Address the patient's main concerns first
- Reassure the patient that he is not having a heart attack and it is only a panic attack

Reassurance

You can reassure him by saying that:

- A person with a panic attack might think that he or she is having a heart attack. This is because some of the symptoms of a panic attack are also experienced during a heart attack (e.g. chest pain).

- It is therefore understandable that a person who is having a panic attack may think he or she is having a heart attack. If chest pain is recurrent or long-lasting, it is wise to have a thorough medical investigation to rule out the presence of heart disease. If heart disease is not present then it is unlikely that subsequent chest pain is caused by a heart attack.

- Heart disease does NOT cause panic attacks and panic attacks do NOT cause heart disease.

- Generally, if an individual who is prone to panic attacks experiences another similar attack, it is probably best for him or her to sit quietly and use the slow breathing exercise for about five to ten minutes. It may also be helpful for the individual to ask himself or herself, 'Did I die or have a heart attack last time I experienced these symptoms?'. However, if pain is still present after ten minutes of slow breathing, the individual is advised to seek medical advice.

What happens during a panic attack and when does this occur?

Panic disorder involves recurrent and sometimes unpredictable attacks of anxiety or panic. The attacks start suddenly, are extremely distressing, and last for a few minutes, sometimes longer. In panic disorder the attacks are not restricted to specific circumstances but may occur in any situation. These attacks may be followed by persistent concern about having another panic attack.

Panic attacks are defined by a sudden onset of intense apprehension, fear (or) terror accompanied by physical symptoms such as:

- difficulty in breathing

- dizziness

- palpitations

- chest pains

- shaking

- sweating

- tingling sensations

- jelly legs

- butterflies in stomach

- feelings of unreality

- fear of dying, losing control (or) going mad

During a panic attack individuals will generally try to flee from the particular situation in the hope that the panic will stop, or else they may seek help in case they collapse, have a heart attack, or go crazy.

What is the panic response?

When we are exposed to a physical threat, our bodies automatically respond so that we are able to defend ourselves or escape from a threatening situation. This response, also known as the 'flight-or-fight' response, involves activity in our nervous system. We become more alert, our heart beat speeds up, the muscles get tense and so ready for action, sweating increases to cool the body, and we breathe very fast in order to get more oxygen to our muscles, to be able to run away or fight.

In these situations, when our rate of breathing increases, we tend to over-breathe or hyperventilate. This hyperventilation causes a number of physical sensations including feelings of dizziness, breathlessness, or pains in the chest.

Consequently we breathe out carbon dioxide; this makes the level in our body low and produces strange physical sensations like dizziness, tingling in our hands and feet, pains in the chest and breathlessness. When people feel breathless, they breathe faster and this will make your symptoms worse. It is important to realise that these feelings are part of the physical response to threat and are not a sign that you have some physical disease. These symptoms do not mean that you will die, go crazy, or lose control. However, because they are part of a stress response, it may be useful for you to look at your life and try to think about what might be troubling you and adding to your stress at the moment.

What happens during hyperventilation?

When you become anxious you set off an emergency or alarm reaction which leads to an increase in the speed and depth of breathing. This over-breathing, also called 'hyperventilation', may lead to the following symptoms:

- **In the brain** it causes dizziness, light-headedness, confusion, breathlessness, blurred vision and feelings of unreality.

- **In the body** it causes an increase in heartbeat to pump more blood around, numbness and tingling in the hands and feet, cold clammy hands, stiffness in the muscles, muscle twitching or cramps and irregular heartbeats. People who over-breathe often tend to breathe from their chest rather than from their diaphragm. As the chest muscles are not made for breathing, these muscles tend to become tired and tense. Thus individuals can experience symptoms of chest tightness or even severe chest pains.

How can we prevent and control hyperventilation?

The first step in preventing and controlling hyperventilation is to recognise *how* and *when* hyperventilation occurs. Many people who panic show some signs of hyperventilation. Hyperventilation may act as the *initial cue* which causes an individual to panic.

In order to reduce the symptoms of hyperventilation it will be necessary to increase and steady the level of carbon dioxide in the blood. One way of achieving increased levels of carbon dioxide is by breathing into a paper bag. This method is simple and effective; however, it may not always be convenient or socially appropriate to pull out a paper bag in a public place!

An alternative method which is less obvious to other people and which will help the individual reduce habitual over-breathing is the slow breathing exercise. Here the individual is instructed to *breathe in* and hold his or her breath, and then instructed to breathe slowly out, saying the word relax to themselves in a calm, soothing manner every time they breathe out. This should be repeated in cycles until all the symptoms of over-breathing have gone.

If individuals follow this exercise as soon as they notice the first signs of over-breathing, the symptoms should subside within a minute or two and panic attacks will hopefully be avoided. The more frequently individuals practise this slow breathing exercise, the better they will become at using slow breathing to prevent anxiety from escalating.

What to do next?

It is very likely that you will be more able to manage panic attacks in the future if:

- You recognise that the symptoms are harmless
- You remember to use the slow breathing exercise when you get anxious
- You learn how to relax and manage your stress more effectively.
- **Note:** It is worth mentioning at the end about information leaflets, fact sheets and other information available in books and on the Internet.

MINI-MENTAL STATE EXAMINATION

Task: Perform the MMSE on Mr White, an elderly person who presented himself to the A&E in a confused state.

The points to be covered are:

- Temporal orientation

- Spatial orientation

- Registration

- Attention, concentration

- Recall

- Naming

- Repetition

- Comprehension

- Reading

- Writing

- Drawing/copying.

Suggested approach

- Greet and introduce yourself

- Purpose of visit should be explained

- Obtain permission before you proceed

- Address whether there are any major concerns

- Check the patient's ability to hear, see and understand you

Max. score	Score	
		Orientation
5	( )	What is the (year), (season), (month), (date), (day).
5	( )	Where are we: (country, county, city/town, building name, floor of the building)
		Registration
3	( )	Ask if you can test the individual's memory. Name 3 objects (e.g. apple, table, penny) taking one second to say each one. Then ask the individual to repeat the names of all three objects. Give one point for each correct answer. After this, repeat the object names until all three are learned – up to 6 trials).

Max. score	Score	
		Attention and calculation
5	( )	Spell 'world' backwards. Give 1 point for each letter that is in the right order DLROW = 5, DLORW = 3). Alternatively, do serial 7s. Ask the individual to count backwards from 100 in blocks of 7 (93, 86, 79, 72, 65). Stop after 5 subtractions. Give one point for each correct answer. If one answer is incorrect (e.g. 92) but the following answer is 7 less than the previous answer (i.e. 85), count the second answer as being correct.
		Recall
3	( )	Ask for the 3 objects repeated above. Give 1 point for each correct object. (Recall should be tested five minutes after presenting the words).
		Language
2	( )	Point to a pencil and ask the individual to name this object (1 point). Do the same with a wrist-watch (1 point).
1	( )	Ask the individual to repeat the following: 'No ifs, ands or buts' (1 point). You may repeat the phrase if the individual has difficulty hearing or understanding you, up to a maximum of five times, but the score should be based only on the first attempt to repeat the phrase.
3	( )	Give the individual a piece of blank white paper and ask him or her to follow a 3-stage command. 'Take the paper in your right hand, fold it in half and put it on the floor' (1 point for each part correctly followed). Give only one trial.
1	( )	Show the individual the 'CLOSE YOUR EYES' message. Ask him or her to read the message and do what it says (give 1 point if the individual actually closes his or her eyes).
1	( )	Ask the individual to write a sentence on a blank piece of paper. The sentence must contain a subject and a verb, and must be sensible. Punctuation and grammar are not important (1 point).
1	( )	Show the individual the intersecting pentagons and ask him or her to copy the design exactly as it is (1 point). All 10 angles need to be present and the two shapes must intersect to score 1 point. Tremor and rotation are ignored.

Total score = ...

■ **Thank the patient for their co-operation**

CRANIAL NERVES EXAMINATION

Task: Examine cranial nerves 1–12 on this patient except for testing of the corneal reflex and fundoscopy.

Suggested approach

- Greet and introduce yourself
- Purpose of visit should be explained
- Obtain permission before you proceed
- Address any major concerns expressed
- Brief history of sight, smell, taste and hearing

1st Cranial nerve

Has he smelled his coffee this morning?

2nd Cranial nerve

To check for visual acuity

- Sit in front of the patient. Ask him to remove his glasses if wearing any.

  a. Check one eye at a time by asking to close other eye. Do the test by finger counting method.

  Or

  b. A near vision chart is provided. Ask the patient to read sections of print from a distance of 30 cm. The smallest size that can be read is recorded (e.g. N6)

To check for field of vision

- Mapping visual fields

Be at the same eye level with the patient. Ask the patient to cover their right eye with their right hand, and cover your left eye with your left hand, and then ask the patient to look in your eye without moving their head. Move your finger to check peripheral fields.

Colour vision

Not essential.

Pupils

- **Direct and consensual reflexes:** A bright light is shone into one eye and the reaction of both pupils (direct and consensual reflexes) is noted. Before you flash the light make sure you tell the patient that you will be shining a bright light in his eyes which may cause a bit of discomfort.

- **Accommodation reflex:** The patient is asked to look into the distance and then at a finger positioned 10 cm directly in front of his/her nose. The pupils are examined as the patient attempts to focus on the finger and the reaction of the pupils to accommodation are noted.

Tell the examiner that ideally you would like to perform **fundoscopy.**

3rd, 4th and 6th Nerve

Ask patient to look into your eyes and to follow your moving finger without moving his head. Describe the letter H with your finger, beginning at the centre of the horizontal line, go to left then up and down, bring the finger back to opposite side and do the same. The patient is asked to report any double vision. Watch for nystagmus.

5th Cranial nerve

Sensory part
Check superficial sensation on various parts of the face with a cotton swab in all three dermatomes alternating both sides. Ask the patient to close his eyes before you proceed and to answer YES when he feels the swab.

Motor part

- Check the **muscles of mastication.**

- Ask to clench the teeth. Then feel for masseters and temporalis.

- The patient is asked to open the mouth against resistance from your hand, which should be placed firmly under the patient's chin.

- You have been asked to ignore the jaw jerk and corneal reflexes.

7th Cranial nerve

Sensory part

- Did you *taste* your breakfast this morning?

Motor part

- Can you show me your teeth please?

- Ask him to shut his eyes tightly while you try to open them gently.

- The motor part is also tested by asking the patient to raise his eyebrows, blow out his cheeks, and purse his lips tightly.

8th Cranial nerve (Vestibulocochlear)

Test hearing sensitivity to a whispered sound or a ticking wristwatch. If there is no problem in hearing inform the patient that you'd like to conduct detailed hearing tests, once you've tested the other nerves.

9th and 10th Cranial nerve

- Request him to open his mouth and ask him to say 'AAAHHH' loudly; comment on soft palate and uvulary movement.
- You have been asked to ignore the gag reflex.

11th Cranial nerve

- Ask the patient to shrug shoulders against resistance.
- Ask the patient to turn his head in both directions against resistance.

12th Cranial nerve

- Ask him to open his mouth and show his tongue and look for any deviation, wasting or tremors.
- Inspect the tongue as it lies on the floor of the mouth, noting any wasting, fasciculation and involuntary movement.
- The patient is then asked to stick out the tongue and move it from side to side.
- State whether examination is normal or not and what you would be doing next.
- Thank the patient and the examiner.

FUNDOSCOPY

Task: To perform an ophthalmoscopic examination on this 45-year-old gentleman and describe your findings and interpretation to the examiner.

What is expected?

- Clear instructions prior to performing an ophthalmoscopic examination
- Appropriate use of ophthalmoscope
- Findings
- Diagnosis

Suggested approach

- Greet the patient and introduce yourself
- Confirm if you have to address the examiner or the patient
- Purpose of visit should be explained
- Obtain permission before you proceed.

Explain that:

- You have to look into the back of his eyes using this light.
- You have to do it with the light in the room switched off.
- The light can be uncomfortable.
- You will have to come so close to the patient that your face may touch his. Get the patient's permission.
- Ensure that the ophthalmoscope is working. Turn it on. Check the light.
- Ask the patient to remove his glasses and look at an object at a distance and at eye level, and to blink and breathe normally.
- Either keep your own glasses/lenses or remove your glasses/lenses and dial up the appropriate lens for your refractive error; – lenses for myopia and + lenses for hypermetropia.
- Stand or sit on the side to be examined at 1 metre from the patient and with eyes level with the patient's. Ask the patient to stare at a fixed point in the distance.
- With the right hand holding the ophthalmoscope, approach the patient's right side at an angle of about 15°, nasally and inwards and at

a distance of 30 cm. Ensure that you use your right eye to examine the patient's right eye and your left eye to examine the patient's left eye.

- Consider your eye and the ophthalmoscope functioning as a single unit. Bring your eye slowly towards the patient's eye until you are as close as possible without touching the eyelashes.

- The back of the patient's eye should be in focus.

- Look systematically, start with the lens, then vitreous, followed by the disc, vessels in the centre, in each quadrant and then the macula.

- When the retina is in focus, follow a blood vessel to the optic disc. The optic disc is slightly pink with sharp borders and a central cup. Look at the four arteries and the accompanying veins, especially where they cross each other. Look for pallor, swelling, new vessel formation, exudates and haemorrhages.

- Locate any abnormality as though the fundus is a clock with the disc at the centre. The diameter of the disc (1.5 mm) is used as the unit of measurement. For example, hard exudates at 4, 6 and 9 o'clock, 2–3 disc diameters from the disc.

- Look at the macula by asking the patient to look directly at the light and using a narrow beam.

Examine both eyes.

The findings should be given in the same order as the examination. Even if the diagnosis is obvious, first inform the findings, and then give the diagnosis.

■ Thank the patient and thank the examiner.

The common slides that are usually kept in the examination are:

1. Normal fundus

2. Papilloedema

3. Diabetic retinopathy

4. Hypertensive retinopathy.

Findings

1. Papilloedema

- The swelling of the disc is called papilloedema

- The optic disc is swollen and pink

- The disc margins are blurred

- The cup is lost

- The retinal arteries and veins of the disc are not clear
- There are congested veins and haemorrhages
- Papilloedema is usually bilateral.

Causes: Malignant hypertension, increased intracranial pressure, cerebral oedema, optic nerve tumours etc.

2. Diabetic retinopathy

Proliferative stage

- Dot (capillary microaneurysms) and blot haemorrhages (leakage of blood into deeper layers of retina).
- Hard exudates (bright yellowish white colour and irregular in outline).
- Tortuous and congested veins.
- New vessel formation near the optic disc.

Hint: If you see yellowish white, glossy, irregular spots, they are hard exudates found in diabetic retinopathy.

3. Hypertensive retinopathy

- Thickening of the arteriolar walls lead to narrowing of the arteriolar blood column, resulting in 'copper-wiring' of arterioles.
- The tortuous and thick walled arterioles compress the narrowed veins at crossings, resulting in venous nipping.
- There may be flame shaped haemorrhages, and soft (cotton wool exudates) and papilloedema.

Hypertensive retinopathy (Keith–Wagener classification)

Grade 1: Tortuosity of the retinal arteries with increased reflectiveness (silver wiring).

Grade 2: Grade 1 plus AV nipping (thickened retinal arteries pass over the retinal veins).

Grade 3: Grade 2 plus flame shaped haemorrhages and soft ('cotton wool') exudates due to small infarcts.

Grade 4: Grade 3 plus papilloedema.

EXTRAPYRAMIDAL SIDE EFFECTS – PHYSICAL EXAMINATION

Task: Mr White has been diagnosed as having paranoid schizophrenia and has been started on one of the conventional antipsychotics. However, he is complaining of stiffness in his arms and legs. Examine him for extrapyramidal signs.

Suggested approach

- Greet the patient and introduce yourself

- Address the patient's concerns first

- Ask the patient briefly about any abnormal movements like slowness, stiffness, shakiness, feeling of inner restlessness and any other body movements which bother the patient

- Explain briefly what you are going to do and ask for consent

- Ensure that the patient knows that during this examination you will be testing his hands, legs, and mouth and that you will make him walk to observe his gait

1. Observe the patient at rest for a few seconds.

2. Ask the patient whether there is anything in his or her mouth and, if so, to remove it.

3. Ask if he or she wears dentures. Ask whether teeth or dentures bother the patient now.

4. Ask whether the patient notices any movements in his or her mouth, face, hands, or feet. If yes, ask the patient to describe them and to indicate to what extent they bother the patient.

5. Ask the patient to open his or her mouth. (Observe the tongue at rest within the mouth.) Do this twice.

6. Ask the patient to protrude his or her tongue. (Observe abnormalities of tongue movement.) Do this twice.

7. Have the patient sit in chair with hands on knees, legs slightly apart and feet flat on floor. (Look at the entire body for movements while the patient is in this position. Observe for 15 seconds.)

8. Ask the patient to sit with hands hanging unsupported – if male, between his legs, if female and wearing a dress, hanging over her knees. (Observe hands and other body areas for at least 15 seconds.)

9. Ask the patient to tap his or her thumb with each finger as rapidly as possible for 10 to 15 seconds, first with right hand, then with left hand. (Observe facial, hand and leg movements.)

10. Flex and extend the patient's left and right arms, one at a time.

11. Ask the patient to stand up. (Observe the patient (15 seconds). Observe all body areas again, hip included.)

12. Ask the patient to extend both arms out in front, palms down. (Observe trunk, legs, and mouth.)

13. Have the patient walk a few paces, turn, and walk back to the chair. (Observe hands and gait.) Do this twice.

- Give a brief report of your findings and thank the patient and the examiner.

FRONTAL LOBE FUNCTION TESTING

Task: Assess the frontal lobe functions for this 65-year-old gentleman with memory problems.

Suggested approach

- Greet the patient and introduce yourself
- Explain briefly what you are going to do and ask for consent

Frontal executive function tests

1. Assessment of verbal fluency

Patient is asked to name as many words as possible beginning with either the letters 'F, A or S'. (Ideally all three ought to be tested) in one minute.

Alternatively you can use a category (name as many animals as possible in one minute). Normal subjects should produce at least 15 words for each letter.

2. Assessment of abstraction

Proverb interpretation
Ask the patient the meaning of two common proverbs:

Example 1: Too many cooks spoil the broth

Example 2: A stitch in time saves nine.

Similarities
The patient is asked to explain the similarities between things (use things that are routinely used).

Example:

a. Table and chair

b. Apple and orange.

3. Co-ordinated movements (tests response inhibition and set shifting)

Alternate sequence
An alternative sequence is shown to the patient and they are asked to copy it.

Go-no-go test

Ask the patient to place a hand on the table and to raise one finger in response to a single tap, while holding still in response to two taps. You tap on the undersurface of the table to avoid giving visual cues.

Luria three-step task

A sequence of hand positions is demonstrated (fist–edge–palm) five times and the patient is asked to repeat it. Check for primitive reflexes such as grasp reflex and palmomental reflex.

Thank the patient and the examiner.

ECG RECORDING

Task: You have been asked to perform a routine ECG on this 'patient'. Explain the procedure as you would to a real patient and place the ECG electrodes on the manikin. Provide a brief report to the examiner on the ECG trace provided.

What is expected?

- Knowledge of placement of the ECG leads
- Information to be given to the patient about the procedure
- Reporting an ECG trace.

Suggested approach

- Greet the 'patient' and introduce yourself
- Explain briefly what you are going to do and take consent
- For example, 'Mr G, I have been asked to do a routine ECG for you'
- This involves me placing some electrodes on your chest, arms and leg
- I'll be connecting these leads to a machine, which will record the electrical activity of your heart, which is the ECG trace
- This is a painless, non-invasive procedure taking about 5 minutes
- Reassure him that this procedure does not involve passing electric current through him, and the procedure itself causes minimal discomfort
- I hope you have no objections to my recording your ECG
- Reassure the 'patient' that the procedure will be stopped if he or she is uncomfortable at any stage.

Positions of limb leads and chest leads

The standard chest lead positions are:

- V1 – Fourth intercostal space, right sternal edge
- V2 – Fourth intercostal space, left sternal edge
- V4 – Fifth intercostal space in the mid-clavicular line
- V3 – Half way between the second and fourth electrodes
- V5 – Fifth intercostal space in the anterior axillary line
- V6 – In line with V5 in the mid axillary line.

The limb lead positions are:

- One on each arm, on the palmar aspect of the wrists
- One on either ankle, on the medial side.

  1. Attach the limb leads to all four limbs, using contact gel under each electrode.

  2. Ensure good contact with the skin.

  3. Switch on the machine and make the recording. Once completed, dispose of the electrode pads and waste appropriately.

Usually a manikin with clear bony markings is provided, so it requires a correct identification of the intercostal space.

- Thank the 'patient' for his co-operation.

INTERPRETATION OF ECG

Task: Comment on the routine ECG tracing of a 50-year-old person with a history of paranoid schizophrenia being treated with an antipsychotic drug. Comment on the ECG.

Comment on the following:

- Rate
- Rhythm
- Regularity
- Axis
- P wave
- PR interval
- QRS complex
- Q waves
- ST segment
- T wave
- QT interval
- Abnormalities
- Opinion
- Management plan.

Comment on the following:

Rate
Divide 300 by the number of large squares between each QRS complex. (Or) between two RR intervals.

Rhythm
If a P wave is seen, then it is a sinus rhythm. Otherwise it is a non-sinus rhythm.

Regularity
This can be regular or irregular. To assess rhythm, lay a card along an ECG and mark the position of three successive R waves. Slide the card back and forth to check that all the intervals are the same.

Axis

- The normal axis lies between −30° and +90°.

- If the QRS complexes in leads I and II are predominantly positive, the axis is normal.

- Left axis deviation exists if lead I is positive, and both leads II and aVF are negative.

- Right axis deviation occurs if lead I is negative, and leads II and aVF are positive.

P wave
This is caused by depolarisation of the atria. Normal height and width are less than 2.5 mm, and 0.11 s respectively in lead II. Comment on whether it is too wide, or too tall.

PR interval
The range is 0.12 to 0.20 s, or 3 to 5 small squares. This should be less than 5 small squares, or else it is prolonged.

QRS complex
The QRS complex represents ventricular depolarisation. Its duration is less than 0.12 seconds, or less than 3 small squares. If more than 0.12 s, a conduction defect is likely.

Q waves
These are pathological if they are more than 25% of the height of the following R wave, and more than 0.04 seconds wide (1 small square).

ST segment
This is normally isoelectric (flat). It can become elevated acutely in myocardial infarction or pericarditis. ST depression occurs in several conditions including myocardial ischaemia and left ventricular hypertrophy.

ST elevation is significant if there are >1 mm elevation in limb leads and > 2 mm elevation in chest leads.

T wave
The T wave represents ventricular repolarisation. T wave inversion in leads I, II, or V 4–6 is usually abnormal. Peaked T waves can occur in hyperkalemia. T wave can be flattened in hypokalemia.

QT interval
This is the interval between the beginning of the QRS complex and the end of the T wave. It varies with heart rate, and so must be corrected – the QTc, or corrected QT interval. To calculate the QTc, divide the QT interval by the square root of the preceding R-R interval (the latter is the interval between

the R waves of two successive QRS complexes). It should be less than 0.42 seconds.

- Corrected QTc = QT/square root of RR interval in seconds.
- Corrected QTc should be approximately 2 large squares.

ECG interpretation

The abnormalities would usually be very evident, so think of common things.

If you can't make out any abnormality, then report the findings as above and then mention whether you think the ECG is normal or abnormal.

ECT – ELECTRODE PLACEMENT

Task: You are requested to administer ECT to Mrs Dorothy Brown who has consented to the procedure. Proceed to administer ECT to the manikin, explaining the steps you take to the examiner. Assume that the appropriate dose has been set and indicate the electrode placement for unilateral and bilateral ECT administration. Using the strip of EEG provided, indicate the different phases of the seizure.

What is expected?

- Knowledge of ECT administration procedures
- Correct electrode placement
- EEG interpretation.

There is no need to speak to the manikin, but you are expected to run through the steps with the examiner.

Suggested approach

- Greet and introduce yourself.
- Obtain permission before you proceed.
- Check that it is the correct 'patient', by cross-check in the file with the identification wrist tag.
- Check documentation to see that she has consented and ECT consent form has been duly signed, or if on a section of the Mental Health Act, appropriate forms have been filled out.
- Ask for consent again and briefly explain the procedure.
- Check that the pre-ECT form has been filled in, with emphasis on nil by mouth for at least 6 hours prior to ECT, physical examination has been done prior to ECT, and anaesthetic opinion obtained.
- Check the medical notes to ensure that the psychiatric team has seen her after the last treatment to record progress and any adverse effects of ECT (if any).
- Check the treatment card to check for current medications.

Electrode positions

Bilateral: 4 cm above the midpoint of the line between external auditory meatus and the lateral angle of the eye.

Unilateral: First electrode is placed on the nondominant side, 4 cm above the midpoint of the line between external angle of the eye and the external auditory meatus. The second electrode is placed 10 cm above the first, vertically above the meatus on the same side.

EEG interpretation

Look for the stimulus on the EEG record. The EEG usually develops patterned sequences consisting of high voltage sharp waves and spikes, followed by rhythmic slow waves that end abruptly in a well-defined endpoint.

- comment on your findings to the examiner

- make sure that you have documented the current used, type and duration of seizures, any complications that arose, in the medical notes and on the ECT form.

- thank the examiner at the end and leave the station.

CARDIOPULMONARY RESUSCITATION

Task: Perform CPR on this collapsed patient in your ward.

Usually the task comes as 'Please provide BLS to this patient who has been found collapsed in the ward (or on the road)'.

This is a strictly dummy station and here there is no need to identify the patient or introduce yourself to the patient.

Please follow the steps in strict order

1. Is it safe to approach? Is there any trauma?

2. After assuming that there is no trauma and the patient is safe, go near the manikin. Shake him by his shoulders and ask loudly at the same time – 'Hello, hello, can you hear me?' or 'Are you OK?'

3. If no response, shout for help – 'Help, Help!' Often the dummies in this station are clad with jumpers or other clothes, so remember to undress the dummy above the waist.

4. Bend down by the side of the manikin's face and **look, listen and feel** for 10 seconds.

5. Check for a **patent airway** to rule out any foreign body, secretions, etc. If the airways are clear, tilt head, lift chin.

6. **Listen and feel** for any effort at breathing.

7. If there are no signs of breathing, activate the **emergency alarm system**.

8. Come back to the patient and give **two effective rescue breaths** – maintain the head tilt, chin lift position and then pinch the nose and purse your lips tightly on the manikin's lips. Blow as forcefully as possible while keeping an eye on the chest expansion. If there is no chest expansion, then either your technique is wrong or the airway is not open.

   Check the airways again and give a further tilt to the head. An effective rescue breath is approximately 500 ml of air with adequate chest expansion.

9. Feel the **peripheral pulses** – the most obvious peripheral pulse is the carotid. Check the pulsation for 10 seconds.

10. If absent, patient will need cardiac compressions. Put the heel of the hand 2 cm above xiphisternum (trace sternum with one hand and subcostal margins with the other and locate xiphisternum at their junction) and place the other hand on top locking the fingers and give **15 chest compressions** (at the rate of 100/min).

11. Repeat the same cycle (**2 breaths: 15 chest compressions**) until:

    a. patient responds

    b. help arrives

    c. or you are exhausted.

12. Once the patient is responsive, put him in the left lateral position, i.e. the **recovery position**.
    A little modification is needed for some special situations such as:

    ● in cases of trauma, we do not tilt the head in case the cervical spine is injured. Instead we give a jaw thrust to open the airway.

    ● with children, in cases of drowning and primary respiratory failure, continue rescue breaths for one minute and if still unresponsive, then activate the alarm system. This is because in all of above if respiratory arrest is reversed, the patient will not need cardiac resuscitation.

RAPID TRANQUILLISATION

Task: Mr Jason Deal is a 28-year-old gentleman admitted to the acute psychiatric ward in a very disturbed state. He was agitated, restless, distressed, complained of hearing voices instructing to kill him or others. He shouted at the ward staff and other patients and remained quite intimidating.

You are the psychiatric SHO on call and they bleeped you to come and assess the patient. The staff are concerned about him and want medication to be prescribed to calm him down. How will you manage the situation?

Acutely disturbed or violent behaviour

Management of an acutely disturbed or violent patient is one of the common clinical scenarios that we face in psychiatric wards. So this can be asked as a separate station.

Acute behavioural disturbance can occur in the context of psychiatric illness, physical illness, substance abuse or personality disorder. Psychotic symptoms are common and the patient may be aggressive towards others, secondary to persecutory delusions or auditory, visual or tactile hallucinations.

Plans for the management of individual patients should ideally be made in advance. The aim is to prevent disturbed behaviour and reduce risk of violence. Nursing interventions (de-escalation, time out), increased nursing levels, transfer of the patient to a psychiatric intensive care unit (PICU) or pharmacological management are all options that may be employed.

In the examination, the steps for rapid tranquillisation (RT) can be asked as a series of questions by the consultant (step 1 to step 5, possible complications and remedial measures).

In an emergency situation:

Step 1

- De-escalation, time out, placement, etc., as appropriate.

Step 2

Offer oral treatment:

- Haloperidol 5 mg with or without lorazepam 1–2 mg or

- Olanzapine 10 mg with or without lorazepam 1–2 mg or

- Risperidone 1–2 mg with or without lorazepam 1–2 mg.

Repeat every 45–60 minutes. Go to step 3 if three doses fail.

Step 3

Consider consultation with senior colleague.

Consider IM treatment. From this point onwards, review the patient's legal status. The requirement for enforced IM medication in informed patients should prompt the use of the Mental Health Act.

- Haloperidol 5 mg with or without lorazepam 1–2 mg or

- Olanzapine 5–10 mg with or without lorazepam 1–2 mg.

(IM olanzapine will be available shortly)

Repeat up to 3 times at 30 minute intervals, if insufficient effect.

Have flumazenil available to reverse the effects of lorazepam. (Monitor respiratory rate – give flumazenil if rate falls below 10/min.)

- Promethazine 50 mg IM is an alternative in benzodiazepine tolerant patients. Promethazine has a slow onset of action but is often an effective sedative. Dilution is not required before IM injection. May be repeated up to a maximum 100 mg/day. Wait 1–2 hours after injection to assess response.

Step 4

Consider consultation with senior colleague.

Consider IV treatment.

- Diazepam 10 mg over at least 5 minutes.

- Repeat after 5–10 minutes if insufficient effect (up to three times).

Use Diazemuls to avoid injection site reactions. IV therapy may be used instead of IM when a very rapid effect is required. IV therapy also ensures near immediate delivery of the drug to its site of action and effectively avoids the danger of inadvertent accumulation of slowly absorbed IM doses. Note also that IV doses can be repeated after only 5–10 minutes if no effect is observed.

Have flumazenil available to reverse the effects of diazepam. (Monitor respiratory rate – give flumazenil if rate falls below 10/min.)

Step 5

Seek expert advice.

- Amylobarbitone 250 mg IM or paraldehyde 5–10 ml IM are options.

Amylobarbitone is a powerful respiratory depressant with no pharmacological antagonist. Have facilities for mechanical ventilation available. Paraldehyde is now used extremely rarely and is difficult to obtain. It should be used when all else has failed. In many cases, ECT may be more appropriate.

Very few episodes of RT should reach this point.

Questions

What are the aims of rapid tranquillisation?

The aims of rapid tranquillisation are threefold:

1. To reduce suffering for the patient: psychological or physical (through self-harm or accidents).

2. To reduce risk of harm to others by maintaining a safe environment.

3. To do no harm (by prescribing safe regimes and monitoring physical health).

How will you monitor a patient after parenteral drug administration?

After any parenteral drug administration monitor as follows:

- Temperature
- Pulse
- Blood pressure
- Respiratory rate.

Every 5–10 minutes for one hour, then half-hourly until patient is ambulatory.

Remedial measures in rapid tranquillisation

Problem 1: Acute dystonia (including oculogyric crises)

- **Remedial measures:**

Give procyclidine 5–10 mg IM or IV, or benzatropine 1–2 mg IM.

Problem 2: Reduced respiratory rate (less than 10/min) or oxygen saturation less than 90%

- **Remedial measures:**
    a. Give oxygen
    b. Raise legs
    c. Ensure the patient is not lying facing down
    d. Give flumazenil, if benzodiazepine-induced respiratory depression suspected
    e. If induced by any other sedative agent: ventilate mechanically.

Problem 3: Irregular or slow pulse (less than 50/min)

- **Remedial measures:**

Refer to specialist medical care immediately.

Problem 4: Fall in blood pressure (>30 mmHg orthostatic drop or <50 mmHg diastolic)

- **Remedial measures:**

    a. Lie patient flat, tilt bed towards head

    b. Monitor closely.

Problem 5: Increased temperature

- **Remedial measures:**

    a. Withhold antipsychotics: (risk of NMS and perhaps arrhythmias)

    b. Check creatinine kinase urgently.

Other useful points

1. Choice depends on current treatment. If the patient is established on antipsychotics, lorazepam may be used alone. If the patient uses street drugs or is already receiving benzodiazepines regularly, an antipsychotic may be used alone. For the majority of patients, the best response will be obtained with a combination of an antipsychotic and lorazepam.

2. Ensure that potential anticholinergics are available. Procyclidine 5–10 mg IM or benzatropine 1–2 mg IM may be required to reverse acute dystonic reactions.

3. Proceed with caution with the very young and elderly and those with pre-existing brain damage or impulse control problems as disinhibition reactions are more likely.

4. If the patient is asleep or unconscious, the use of pulse oximetry to continuously measure oxygen saturation is desirable.

5. A nurse should remain with the patient until they are ambulatory again.

6. ECG and haematological monitoring are also strongly recommended when parenteral antipsychotics are given, especially when higher doses are used.

EXAMINATION OF THYROID GLAND

Task: Mrs Smith suffers from bipolar affective disorder. She is currently on lithium 800 mg and over the last six months she has been feeling increasingly tired and lethargic. Carry out an examination to assess the patient for thyroid disorder.

Examination of thyroid gland

- Greet and introduce yourself
- Purpose of visit should be explained
- Obtain permission before you proceed
- Build rapport and address the patient's main concerns
- In the case of female patient, ask for a chaperone

General examination

- Nails – pallor/clubbing/cyanosis
- Hands – sweating/warmth/acropachy/acrocyanosis
- Tremors
- Pulse – rate and rhythm
- Tongue – pallor/cyanosis
- Legs – pretibial myxoedema.

Local examination

- Check the exposure from jaw to the nipple line.

Inspection

Look for

- Any obvious swelling on swallowing and on protrusion of tongue
- Scars, sinuses and erythema
- Any dilated or engorged veins in the neck and on the chest
- Visible pulsations if any.

Palpation

From front
- Confirm findings of inspection

- Feel for the trachea and its displacement if present
- Carotid pulsations: feel one at a time.

From behind

- Lahey's method
- Lower limit of thyroid is checked while the patient is swallowing
- Check for cervical lymphadenopathy.

Percussion

- Only if lower limit of the gland is not palpable (direct percussion on the sternum).

Auscultation

- Check for thyroid and carotid bruit.

Eye signs

- Exophthalmos (from behind)
- Lid retraction and lid lag.

Reflexes

- Ankle jerk.

Elicit clinical symptoms of hyperthyroidism

Symptoms

1. Weight loss despite increased appetite
2. Heat intolerance
3. Sweating
4. Diarrhoea
5. Tremors
6. Irritability
7. Anxiety
8. Emotional lability

9. Frenetic activity

10. Psychosis

11. Itch

12. Oligomenorrhoea

13. Infertility

Signs

- Tachycardia
- Atrial fibrillation
- Warm extremities
- Fine tremors
- Goitre and nodules
- Palmar erythema
- Hair thinning
- Lid lag
- Bulging eyes
- Eye signs

Elicit clinical symptoms of hypothyroidism

Symptoms

1. Tiredness

2. Lethargy

3. Weight gain

4. Constipation

5. Dislike of cold

6. Menorrhagia

7. Hoarse voice

8. Depression

9. Dementia

10. Myalgia

Signs

- Bradycardia
- Dry skin and hair
- Goitre
- Slowly relaxing reflexes
- Congestive cardiac failure
- Non-pitting oedema
- Toad-like face
- Peripheral neuropathy
- Pericardial effusion

SENSORY AND MOTOR EXAMINATION

Task: Perform sensory and motor system examination for this 45-year-old gentleman admitted recently to your ward.

Take care that you have to be *quick, informative and precise* during this examination.

Note: Checking sensory system and motor system for upper limbs and lower limbs can be asked individually as separate stations.

Procedure

- Introduce yourself to the patient

- Confirm the identity of the patient

- Obtain verbal consent from the patient

- Ensure privacy and achieve adequate exposure

- In case of females do not forget to ask for chaperone

- Ask the relevant neurological history such as history of tingling, numbness, heaviness, etc.

- Uncover the limb to be examined with the consent of the patient

General examination

- Nails – pallor, cyanosis, capillary filling and trophic changes

- Hair loss on the limb

- Any obvious joint pathology

- Pulse.

Inspection

- Posture of limb

- Any deformity

- Wasting of limb and fasciculation

- Scars, sinuses, erythema or swelling.

Palpation

- Ask permission before you proceed

- Temperature – compare both the sides
- Limb girth measurement – above and below the joint.

Sensory examination

For this exam purpose you check for:

Dorsal column

Superficial sensation
Test using a cotton swab. The patient should have his eyes closed. The patient should feel the cotton swab on his face or sternum before you proceed.

Vibration sense
Use 128 Hz frequency tuning fork. Tell patient that this is a tuning fork and when you place it on his bony prominences it will feel like a buzz. Usually it is tested on the first metacarpo-phalangial joint for upper limb and first metatarso-phalangial joint for the lower limbs. Here again make the patient feel the tuning fork on his sternum before you proceed and ensure his eyes are closed.

Positional sense
Tested by checking movement of the distal interphalangial joint of the thumb or big toe with eyes closed. If the patient cannot feel the position then check the proximal joints till he feels it. (If he cannot feel moving first distal interphalangial joint, then move the wrist or ankle, if still negative move the elbow or knee joint.)

Lateral column

Pain sensation
Tested here with red-headed pins on the dermatomes. They do not usually allow pain sensation to be tested, but you must mention that ideally you would like to test it.

Temperature
Mention that ideally you would like to test the temperature also.

Motor examination

Check for tone
Ensure that he does not have any joint pain in that limb.

Check power

- For upper limbs: flexors at elbow
- Wrist flexors
- Thumb extensors and opposition
- Interossei with the card test
- Upper limb: quadriceps
- Hamstrings
- Plantar flexion
- Extensors of big toe.

Reflexes

- Upper limb: biceps for C5
- Triceps for C7
- Supinator for C6
- Lower limb: ankle for S1 and check for clonus at the same time
- Knee for L3–4
- Check the plantars last.

Cerebellar signs

- Upper limb: finger–nose test (one test is enough)
- Lower limb: knee–heel test.

Check for gait, posture and involuntary movements.

Conclusion

- For lower limbs – dorsolumbar spine
- For upper limbs – cervical spine
- Make sure the patient is dressed
- Thank the patient and the examiner.

CARDIOVASCULAR EXAMINATION

Task: Examine the cardiovascular system of this 45-year-old gentleman admitted to your ward.

Suggested approach

- Introduce yourself to the patient
- Confirm the identity of the patient
- Obtain verbal consent from the patient
- Ensure privacy and achieve adequate exposure
- In case of females do not forget to ask for chaperone

General examination

- **Nails** – Pallor/clubbing/cyanosis/splinter haemorrhage
- **Palm** – Palmar erythema
- **Pulse** – Rate and rhythm with radial pulse. Volume and character in brachial pulses on both sides
- **Carotids** – Check one at a time
- **Eyes** – Jaundice and pallor
- **Tongue** – Pallor and cyanosis
- **JVP** – Ask the patient to recline at 45° on the couch. Turn his head to the left side and look for any rise of JVP.
- **Oedema** – Ankles. But mention that you would like to look for sacral oedema.

Systemic examination

Inspection

- Apex beat
- Deformity
- Visible pulsation and apex beat
- Redness, scars and sinuses
- Engorged veins.

Palpation

- Remember to ask for permission before touching the patient
- Locate the apex beat and mention its character
- Feel for any thrills
- Parasternal heave.

Percussion is not necessary here.

Auscultation

1. **Apex:** Ask patient to turn to left side. Auscultate first with diaphragm then with bell.

2. **Tricuspid:** Use diaphragm.

3. **Pulmonary:** Use diaphragm. Listen for any splitting of sounds on deep inspiration.

4. **Aortic:** Use diaphragm. Ask patient to lean forward and hold breath in deep expiration.

5. Auscultation of the base of lungs for crepitations.

Mention that you would like to complete the examination by taking **blood pressure** and examine for any **hepatomegaly.**

- **Ask the patient to dress.**
- **Thank the patient and thank the examiner.**

GASTROINTESTINAL EXAMINATION

Task: Examine the gastrointestinal system of this 45-year-old gentleman admitted to your ward.

Procedure

- Introduce yourself to the patient
- Confirm the identity of the patient
- Obtain verbal consent from the patient
- Ensure privacy and achieve adequate exposure
- In case of females do not forget to ask for chaperone
- Ask patient to lower his trousers as often Pfannenstiel's incisions are missed

General examination

- **Nails** – Pallor/clubbing/cyanosis
- **Palm** – Palmar erythema/Dupuytren's contracture/flapping tremors
- **Pulse** – Rate and rhythm
- **Eye** – Jaundice and pallor
- **Tongue** – Pallor, cyanosis and fetor hepaticus
- **Oedema** – Ankle, but mention that you would like to look for sacral oedema
- **Cervical lymphadenopathy** especially Virchow's lymph node
- **Chest** – Gynaecomastia, loss of chest or axillary hair and spider naevi.

Systemic examination

Inspection

- Shape of the abdomen
- Type of respiration
- Position of umbilicus
- Swelling, redness, scars and sinuses in the abdomen

- Visible pulsations in the abdomen
- Caput medusa with other venous engorgement.

Palpation

Palpate abdomen for guarding, rigidity and tenderness.
Feel for any obvious mass.

Palpate organs

1. Liver

2. Spleen

3. Kidneys (bimanual)

4. Test for ascites – fluid thrill.

Percussion

- Liver dullness
- Fluid shift.

Auscultation

- For bowel sounds
- Aortic and renal bruit.

■ Conclude examination by mentioning per rectal examination and hernial orifices.

■ Ask patient to dress and thank the patient and the examiner.

RESPIRATORY SYSTEM EXAMINATION

Task: Examine the respiratory system of this 45-year-old gentleman admitted to your ward.

Procedure

- Introduce yourself to the patient
- Confirm the identity of the patient
- Obtain verbal consent from the patient
- Ensure privacy and achieve adequate exposure
- In case of females do not forget to ask for chaperone

General examination

- **Nails** – Pallor/clubbing/cyanosis
- **Pulse** – Rate, rhythm and volume
- **Eye** – Jaundice and pallor
- **Tongue** – Pallor and cyanosis

Systemic examination

Inspection

1. Movement of the chest
2. Deformity
3. Respiratory rate
4. Respiratory pattern – abdominothoracic or reverse
5. Visible pulsations and apex beat
6. Accessory muscles of respiration
7. Redness, scars, sinuses and engorged veins

Palpation

Remember to ask permission before touching the patient.

a. Tracheal position
Inform the patient that you will be pressing on his airway and it will cause him some discomfort.

b. **Respiratory movements:** To check

- Anterior part: Supramammary and inframammary region

- Posterior: Interscapular and subscapular region

- Lateral: Chest expansion

c. **Tactile vocal fremitus:** Not essential

d. **Apex beat**

Percussion

- Tell patient that you will be tapping on his chest, but won't be hurting him. Tell him to feel free to say stop if this is uncomfortable.

- Areas to be percussed – direct percussion over clavicle then follow same areas of palpation. Do not forget lateral aspect over axilla and posterior aspect.

Auscultation

- Same areas as palpation and percussion

- Mention any **adventitious sounds and basal crepitations**

Vocal resonance

Must be done as tactile vocal fremitus is not tested.

- Conclude that you would ideally check for upper respiratory tract pathologies and cervical lymph nodes. Do not forget to ask patient to dress and thank him and examiner.

ALCOHOL MISUSE – PHYSICAL EXAMINATION

Task: Mr Brown is a 45-year-old gentleman who is a known alcoholic and was admitted earlier this morning because of his heavy alcohol misuse. He has not yet had a physical examination. Given his history, conduct an appropriate physical examination. Explain to the examiners what you are looking for.

Procedure

- Introduce yourself to the patient
- Confirm the identity of the patient
- Obtain verbal consent from the patient
- Ensure privacy and achieve adequate exposure
- In case of females do not forget to ask for chaperone
- **Briefly ask for symptoms of alcohol withdrawal** like tremors, sweating, agitation, restlessness and feeling anxious

Examine the patient from the end of the bed

Look for classical stigmata, such as:

- Jaundice
- Abdominal distension
- Spider naevi mainly on trunk, face and arms
- Caput medusae (dilated veins on the abdominal wall)
- Gynaecomastia.

General examination

Examine skin

Abrasions, bruises, scars suggestive of falls or violence.

Examine hair

Decreased body hair.

Examine face

- Facial redness
- Bilateral parotid enlargement.

Examine eyes

- Icterus
- Pallor
- Check for nystagmus
- Check for lateral gaze palsy.

Examine hands

- Leuconychia
- Clubbing
- Palmar erythema
- Dupuytren's contracture
- Ask patient to bend both hands back, looking for asterixis (flapping tremor).

Systemic examination

Cardiovascular examination

Pulse – tachycardia
Blood pressure – hypertension (raised in heavy alcohol misuse)
Precordial examination and auscultation
Peripheral oedema (heart failure seen with heavy alcohol misuse).

Respiratory examination

Respiratory rate – orthopnoea.

Abdominal examination

- Checks for asymmetry
- Checks for ascites
- Hepatomegaly
- Testicular atrophy (males).

Neurological examination

Motor examination

- **Bulk and tone:** Muscle wasting; cogwheel rigidity (alcoholic pellagra encephalopathy)

- **Power:** Loss of power with heavy drinking; quadriplegia (central pontine myelinosis)

- **Reflexes:** Increased deep tendon reflexes

- **Abnormal movements:**
  Tremor seen in acute alcohol withdrawal (delirium tremens)
  Myoclonus and oppositional hypertonus (alcoholic pellagra, encephalopathy)

- **Co-ordination and gait:** Ataxia (cerebellar damage, Wernicke's syndrome, and Marchiafava–Bignami disease).

Sensory examination

- **Sensation:** Loss of pain sensation in the limbs and trunk (central pontine myelinosis).

Other cortical functions

- Speech – dysarthria (Marchiafava–Bignami disease)

- Vision – loss of visual acuity (optic atrophy)

- Orientation – confusion seen in a variety of alcohol-induced states.

- ■ **Do not forget to ask patient to dress.**

- ■ **Thank the patient and the examiner.**

OPIATE WITHDRAWAL – PHYSICAL EXAMINATION

Task: You are called to see a 29-year-old man with a long history of heroin abuse who presented to the hospital last night. Assess him for opiate withdrawal, explaining to the examiner what you are looking for.

Procedure

- Introduce yourself to the patient
- Confirm the identity of the patient
- Obtain verbal consent from the patient
- Ensure privacy and achieve adequate exposure
- In case of females do not forget to ask for chaperone
- Ask about the following symptoms: craving, arthralgia, myalgia, abdominal cramps, vomiting and diarrhoea
- Observe for signs of withdrawal:

  Agitation

  Anxiety/irritability

  Restlessness (observation during assessment)

  Sweating

  Tremor (observation of outstretched hands).

General examination

Examine skin

- Sweating
- Piloerection (gooseflesh skin, necessary to feel skin)
- Abrasions, bruises, scars suggestive of falls or violence
- Scratch marks
- Look for any signs of dehydration.

Examine eyes

- Dilated pupils

- Watery eyes (lacrimation)
- Icterus.

Examine face

- Rhinorrhoea (not accounted for by cold symptoms or allergies)
- Yawning (observation during assessment).

Examine for:

- Injection sites
- Scars, infection, ulcers, abscesses or other signs of local inflammation.

Examine for:

- Fever (if thermometer not available, candidate should ask)
- Hyperglycaemia – obtain consent to do random blood glucose testing (hyperglycaemia in withdrawals – at least worth mentioning in the exam).

Systemic examination

Cardiovascular examination

- Hyper/hypotension
- Tachycardia
- Murmurs.

Respiratory system examination

- Respiratory rate: tachypnoea
- Any signs of infection in the respiratory tract.

Abdominal examination

- Hepatomegaly
- Splenomegaly.

Neurological examination

- Muscle tone and power – look for muscle wasting
- Reflexes

- Gait and co-ordination
- Peripheral sensation.

■ Do not forget to ask patient to dress. Thank the patient and the examiner.

EATING DISORDER – PHYSICAL EXAMINATION

Task: Miss Pang is an 18-year-old lady who was admitted earlier today because of problems with eating and weight loss. Given her history, please conduct an appropriate physical examination. Explain to the examiners what you are looking for.

Procedure

- Introduce yourself to the patient
- Confirm the identity of the patient
- Obtain verbal consent from the patient
- Ensure privacy and achieve adequate exposure
- In case of females do not forget to ask for chaperone
- Measure patient's weight (if scales available)
- Measure patient's height (if equipment available)

General examination

Examine skin

- Purpuric rash
- Signs of dehydration
- Areas of skin breakdown
- Skin tone – possibility of hypercarotinaemia
- Any signs of infection.

Examine hands and arms

- Palmar creases for pallor
- Look for Lanugo hair (may be seen on arms, but typically on trunk)
- Brittle hair and nails.

Examine hair

Normal secondary sexual hair pattern unaffected.

Examine eyes

Look for pallor.

Cardiovascular examination

- Pulse (bradycardia)
- Blood pressure (hypotension)
- Precordial examination and auscultation
- Peripheral oedema (may be seen).

Respiratory examination

Gastrointestinal examination

- Look in mouth for:
  a. Signs of dehydration
  b. Dental caries
  c. Damaged enamel from vomiting
  d. Incisor damage from self-induced vomiting with fingers
  e. Swollen salivary glands.
- Abdominal distension (constipation, acute gastric dilatation)
- Tenderness over the abdominal area (acute pancreatitis).

Neurological examination

Peripheral neuropathy.

Other test

'Squat test' – ability of patient to rise from squatting position unaided.

- Do not forget to ask the patient to dress.
- Thank the patient and the examiner.

INTERPRETING BLOOD RESULTS: NEUROLEPTIC MALIGNANT SYNDROME

Task: You are asked to see a 29-year-old man who has become increasingly physically unwell over the last 48 hours.

Current medication

1. Zuclopenthixol decanoate 300 mg weekly. He was started on this two weeks previously.

2. Procyclidine 5 mg bid.

Symptoms

He is sweaty, agitated, and a little tremulous.

Blood results

FBC, 15.8; WCC, 17.8; platelets, 387; Na, 144; Cl, 103; K, 3.9; urea, 8.3; creatinine, 102.

Other

Temperature, 38.2°C, BP, 144/100, HR, 109/min.

Questions

1. What is the most likely diagnosis?
2. What are the other symptoms and signs of this condition?
3. What are the risk factors causing this condition?
4. What other investigations would you like to do?
5. How would you manage this condition?
6. What about prescribing antipsychotics in the future?
7. When do you prefer ECT treatment for NMS?

Answers

1. Possible neuroleptic malignant syndrome

2. Signs and symptoms

- **Symptoms:** Fever, diaphoresis, rigidity, confusion, fluctuating consciousness, fluctuating blood pressure, tachycardia

- **Signs:** Elevated creatinine kinase, leukocytosis, altered liver function tests.

3. Risk factors

- High potency typical antipsychotic drugs
- Recent or rapid dose increase of antipsychotics
- Rapid dose reduction
- Abrupt withdrawal of anticholinergic drugs
- Psychosis, organic brain disease, alcoholism, Parkinson's disease
- Hyperthyroidism
- Agitation
- Dehydration.

4. Investigations

- **Blood tests include:**

  a. Creatine phosphokinase (CK) – elevated

  b. Arterial blood gases (looking for metabolic acidosis)

  c. Coagulation screen

  d. Serum iron (has been reported to be low)

- **EEG:** Non-focal generalised slowing on electroencephalography, consistent with encephalopathy, has been reported in over half of NMS cases

- **CT scan**

- **Lumbar puncture.**

Cerebrospinal fluid examinations, sepsis evaluation, brain imaging studies are negative in NMS, and allow for the exclusion of other causes of fever and neurological deterioration.

5. Management

In the psychiatric unit:

  a. Withdraw antipsychotics

  b. Monitor temperature, pulse, BP.

In the medical unit:

- Rehydration.

- Sedation with **benzodiazepines** which are useful in reversing catatonia, are easy to administer, and can be tried initially in most cases.

- Trials of **bromocriptine, amantadine,** or other dopamine agonists may be tried in patients with moderate symptoms of NMS.

- **Dantrolene sodium** appears to be beneficial in cases of NMS involving significant rigidity and hyperthermia. It has been beneficial in rapidly reducing extreme temperature elevations in many cases.

- **Artificial ventilation** if required.

- **L-dopa** and **carbamazepine** have also been used.

- Consider **ECT** for treatment after other interventions have failed.

6. Restarting

- Antipsychotic treatment will be required in most instances and 'antipsychotics rechallenge' is associated with acceptable risk.

- Stop antipsychotics for at least 5 days, preferably longer.

- Allow time for symptoms and signs to resolve completely.

- Begin with very small dose and increase very slowly with close monitoring of temperature, pulse and blood pressure.

- CK monitoring may be used, but is controversial.

- Consider using an antipsychotic structurally unrelated to that associated with NMS or a drug with low dopamine affinity (quetiapine or clozapine).

- Avoid depots and high potency conventional antipsychotics.

7. ECT may be preferred

a. If NMS symptoms are refractory to other measures

b. In patients with prominent catatonic features

c. In patients who develop a residual catatonic state or remain psychotic after NMS has resolved.

SEROTONIN SYNDROME

Task: You are asked to see a 32-year-old man who has been becoming more physically unwell over the last 24 hours. He is not your patient, but you know that his antidepressants have very recently been changed. His symptoms are confusion, restlessness, agitation, sweating and shivering.

1. What is the most likely diagnosis?

2. What other information would you like?

3. What other findings would you look for?

4. How would you manage him?

Answers

1. Serotonin syndrome

2. Important information would include:

a. Previous antidepressants, their dose, and duration of treatment

b. New antidepressants, their dose, and duration of treatment

c. Length of 'washout' period, if any

d. Previous reactions or intolerance to medications.

3. Other findings to look for would include:

a. Fever

b. Tachycardia

c. Myoclonus

d. Hyperreflexia

e. Incoordination

f. Oculogyric crisis

4. Treatment involves: in the Psychiatric unit;

a. Monitoring of physical condition

b. Stopping any serotonergic drugs, especially antidepressants

c. Discussion with medical colleagues and transfer if condition deteriorates

d. Treatment steps in the medical unit may involve:

- Close monitoring of vital signs.

- Proper hydration, i.v. fluids (if necessary)
- Cooling blankets for hyperthermia
- Anticonvulsants for seizures
- Intramuscular chlorpromazine as an antipyretic and sedative agent
- Clonazepam for myoclonus
- Nifedipine for hypertension
- Artificial ventilation for respiratory insufficiency.

INTERPRETING BLOOD RESULTS – EATING DISORDER

Task: A 19-year-old girl is admitted with anorexia nervosa.

Physical findings

Pulse, 56 bpm
BP, 86/62 mmHg
Temperature 36.2°C.

Look at the following blood results.

Haematology		Biochemistry	
Hb	9.3	Sodium	129
WCC	3.5	Potassium	3.2
Platelets	137	Chloride	97
MCV	94.3	Urea	8.5
MCH	Not available	Creatinine	138
Haematocrit	0.28	Calcium	2.01
ESR	2	Magnesium	0.65
		Phosphate	0.63
		Glucose random	3.4
		Creatinine kinase	187

Liver function tests		Thyroid function tests	
AST	47	TSH	0.03
ALT	58	T_4	25.7
Alk Phos	135	T_3	Not available
Bilirubin	25		
GGT	64		
Albumin	35		

Questions

1. Looking at the list of investigations, identify if there are any abnormalities.

2. What investigations would you do routinely in a patient with anorexia nervosa?

3. What are the endocrine changes that can be expected in a patient with anorexia nervosa?

4. What are the metabolic abnormalities and blood changes that can be expected in a patient with anorexia nervosa?

5. What are the cardiac and gastrointestinal complications that can be expected in a patient with anorexia nervosa?

6. What other abnormalities might you expect to find?

7. When would you consider inpatient treatment?

Answers

1. The abnormalities identified include:

- Bradycardia
- Hypotension
- Anaemia
- Leucopenia
- Thrombocytopenia
- Hyponatremia
- Hypokalemia
- Low calcium, phosphate, and magnesium
- Abnormal LFTs
- High T_4 with suppressed TSH.

2. Essential investigations would comprise:

a. FBC

b. U&E

c. Glucose

d. LFTs

e. TFTs

f. Vitamin B and folate levels

g. Serum calcium, magnesium, phosphate

h. ECG.

3. The possible endocrine changes that can be expected are:

- GH (raised)
- Cortisol (positive DST) level raised
- Gonadotrophin levels decreased
- Oestrogens level decreased

- Testosterone level decreased
- T_3 (sick euthyroid syndrome) levels decreased
- Amenorrhoea/loss of libido.

4. The metabolic abnormalities that can be expected are:

- Dehydration
- Hypoglycemia (due to bingeing and purging) and impaired glucose tolerance (due to starvation)
- Deranged LFTs
- Hypercholesterolemia
- Hypokalemia
- Hypoproteinemia
- Plasma amylase (raised)
- lowered calcium, magnesium and phosphate levels

Haematological:

- Normochromic, normocytic, or iron-deficient anaemia
- Leucopenia, with a relative lymphocytosis
- Thrombocytopenia
- Low ESR
- Hypocellular marrow
- Reduced serum complement level.

5. The cardiovascular and gastrointestinal complications include:

Cardiovascular:

- Peripheral oedema
- Congestive cardiac failure
- Bradycardia
- Hypotension
- Decreased heart size
- QT prolongation.

Gastrointestinal:

- Swollen salivary glands
- Dental caries

- Erosion of enamel (vomiting)
- Delayed gastric emptying
- Acute gastric dilations (bulimic episodes, vigorous refeeding, constipation)
- Acute pancreatitis.

6. Other complications of anorexia include:

Neurological:
- EEG abnormalities
- Seizures
- Peripheral neuropathy
- Cerebral oedema.

Renal:
- Acute/chronic renal failure
- Hypokalemic nephropathy
- Proteinuria
- Reduced GFR.

Musculoskeletal:
- Osteoporosis
- Pathological fractures
- Proximal myopathy
- Stunted growth
- Muscle cramps.

Other:
- Hypothermia
- Bacterial infections (TB, staph)
- Lanugo hairs on trunk
- Brittle hair and nails.

6. Inpatient treatment will be considered if:

a. BMI is less than 13.5

b. Severe physical or psychiatric risk

c. Failed outpatient treatment.

SUICIDE RISK ASSESSMENT AND MANAGEMENT

Task: Assess the current risk of suicide in Miss Vicky Smith, a young woman admitted to the medical ward following an overdose.

Suicide risk assessment has usually been asked as a paired station, where in the first station you will be asked to do a risk assessment, and in the next station you have to discuss with the consultant, over the phone, about the assessment done and your further management plan.

Suicide risk assessment:

- Obtain more information about the overdose
- Evaluate the degree of suicidal intent and seriousness of the attempt
- Investigate symptoms of depression/psychosis
- Assess current mental state including suicidal thoughts
- Past history and background information
- Assess coping methods and ability to seek help.

Suggested approach

- Greet and introduce yourself
- Purpose of visit should be explained
- Obtain permission before you proceed
- The patient may be distressed
- Acknowledge her distress
- Allow her to speak freely for the first few moments noting her concerns
- Start with open questions

Step 1: Obtain the following information about the overdose

1. How many tablets were taken?
2. What type of tablets were taken?
3. When was the overdose taken?
4. How was the medication obtained?
5. Where was the patient when she took the overdose?
6. How and by whom was she discovered?

7. How did she reach hospital and who brought her?

8. Did she take anything else with the tablets, for example, alcohol?

9. Why did she take the overdose? (Or)

What was the event leading up to the suicidal act? (Or)

What made her think of harming herself? (Or)

What sorts of things have been worrying her? Examples:

- Conflict in a close relationship
- A major loss or separation
- Family disharmony
- Difficulties at work
- Financial worries/housing
- Health problems
- Redundancy or legal problems.

Step 2: Assessment of the degree of suicidal intent and seriousness of the attempt

A detailed assessment should include evaluation of the characteristics of the attempt:

A. The degree of suicidal intent

- Did the person plan the attempt carefully or was it impulsive?
- Did she take measures to avoid discovery?
- Did she convey her suicidal intent to others?
- Did she leave any suicide note?

Remember 4 Ps:
P – Planning/impulsivity
P – Performance in isolation or in front of others
P – Preparations made prior to the act
P – Precautions to avoid discovery of others.

B. The seriousness of the attempt

- What method was used?
- Did the person understand the consequences of the method she used?
   a. For example, was the person taking an overdose aware of the actions of the drug and did she believe that the dose taken would be fatal?
   b. Did she take all the tablets or did she leave behind a few?

c. What are the problems experienced by the patient currently?

(Please see point 9 in step 1)

Step 3: Explore depressive symptoms (see chapter on assessing depression) and or psychotic symptoms with duration and their impact on current functioning

Step 4: Assess current mental state: mood and hopelessness

- How do you feel in yourself?
- How do you see the future?
- Do you still feel that life is not worth living?

Suicidal thoughts and plans

- Do you still have thoughts of harming yourself in any way?
- What do you think you might do?
- Have you made any plans?
- When are you intending to do it?
- What prevents you from doing it?

Step 5: Past history and background information

- Does she have a past history of suicidal behaviour?
- Does she suffer from a mental illness, for example depression, psychosis, anxiety disorder, borderline personality disorder?
- Is there a history of non-compliance with treatment?
- Does she abuse alcohol or drugs?
- Is there a family history of mental illness, alcohol or substance abuse, violence or suicidal behaviour?

Step 6: Coping methods and ability to seek help

- What were her reactions to previous stresses, failures and losses?
- What does she usually do when there is a problem?
- How does she usually cope?
- With whom does she share her worries?
- How supportive are family and friends?
- Does she get any help?
- In the past, did anyone offer her any help? How did she find it?

Decision making and developing a management plan

Decision making

After the assessment:

1. If she does appear to have a mental illness, which is of the nature and degree that requires hospital treatment or if she is likely to be at risk to herself should she leave hospital at this time, then try to encourage a voluntary admission.

2. If that does not work, it would be appropriate to detain her under Section 5 (2) of the Mental Health Act and you should also let the RMO know that the patient is on Section 5 (2), so that a Mental Health Act assessment can be arranged as soon as possible and detention under Section 2 or 3 can be considered if necessary.

Developing a management plan

When caring for an individual who is recovering from a suicide attempt, it is important to develop a management plan to help the individual get safely through this period of distress.

The general suggestions for this management plan are outlined below.

- Ensure appropriate supervision/hospitalisation for the individual.

- Do not leave the individual alone for any length of time. Family and friends may be able to provide suitable supervision. If the patient is to be admitted to the hospital, increase the level of nursing observation.

- Involve family members in caring for the individual. Encourage a supportive network away from the clinician (e.g. family, friends, and agencies). Help the individual to resolve any immediate conflicts with others.

- Ensure the individual has immediate 24-hour access and support and give the individual a list of contact numbers (e.g. crisis team, extended hours team, general practitioner, hospital, telephone support).

- Remove all means of committing suicide.

- If the individual requires medication, ensure she only has access to a very small amount.

- Conduct a thorough assessment of the individual's situation.

- Neutralise the precipitating problem.

  If you discharge this patient, give a follow-up outpatient appointment with your team in a week's time and make arrangements for one of the members of the community mental health to contact the patient, within the next 24 hours.

PUERPERAL DISORDER – ASSESS RISK

Task: A&E staff asks you to see Miss Williams; a young woman who is 2 weeks postpartum and has presented to the A&E saying there is something wrong with her baby boy. The A&E staff is concerned about her. Do a risk assessment.

Areas to be concentrated upon

- Explore the risk factors
- Assess relationship to the baby
- Assess the mother's mental state
a. Look for depressive symptoms and negative thoughts
b. Look for psychotic symptoms
c. Thoughts of harming herself and the baby
d. Cognitive state and insight
- Relevant history including past psychiatric history, family history and social support.

Suggested approach

- Greet and introduce yourself
- Purpose of visit should be explained
- Obtain permission before you proceed
- The patient may be distressed, confused and paranoid
- Acknowledge her distress
- Allow her to speak freely for the first few moments noting her concerns
- Start with open questions

1. Risk factors

Ask briefly about 4Ps:

- Parity and age
- Planned pregnancy or not?
- Problems during pregnancy and during labour:

    How did you get on generally during the pregnancy?

    Tell me about how the delivery went.

- Partner:

  Are you currently in a relationship?

  How are things between you and your partner/husband?

  Have there been any difficulties since the baby was born?

2. Relationship with the baby

- Please tell me about your baby
- How do you feel about your baby?
- How are you coping with the baby?
- Does he sleep well?
- Does he cry too much?
- Have you been losing your temper with the baby?

Ask questions regarding her anxiety about the wellbeing of the baby and any abnormal ideas about the baby

- Does he have any problems?
- Are you worried/concerned about the baby?
- Do you think there is something wrong with the baby?
- Do you have worrying thoughts about the baby?
- Are you worried that someone might take the baby away?

Ask about depressive symptoms and psychotic symptoms

Tiredness, insomnia, weepiness, irritability, anxiety, paranoid thoughts, hearing voices.

3. Mental state examination

- How do you feel in yourself?
- How do you feel as a mother?
- Do you feel useless or worthless as a mother?
- Do you feel trapped as a mother?
- Do you blame yourself for something you have done or thought?

Risk assessment – explore any thoughts of harming herself or the baby

- Have you thought of doing something to yourself?
- What would you do?
- Do you have any thoughts of harming yourself?

- Do you feel that you need to do something to the baby?
- Can you explain that please?
- Have you heard voices that tell you to harm the baby?

Cognitive functions – look for disorientation to time and place

- Insight
    a. What do you think is the problem?
    b. Do you think you might be unwell?

4. Other relevant history

- Past psychiatric history
- Family history
- Social supports: marital conflict, other stressors
- Any misfortunes like bereavement, the partner's losing his job, housing and money problems, etc.

Note: It is almost impossible to cover all the questions in 7 minutes, but it is a good idea to ask at least three or four questions in each subheading to cover the important aspects and obtain a global pass!

ALCOHOL – PROBLEMS, RISKS AND MOTIVATION

Task: Mr Hughes is a 45-year-old gentleman admitted to the medical ward with gastro-oesophageal reflux disease. Counsel this patient about the risks of excessive alcohol intake and ways to deal with this problem.

Suggested approach

- Greet and introduce yourself

- Purpose of visit should be explained

- Obtain permission before you proceed

- Address his main concerns

- Start with open questions

- **DO NOT TAKE ALCOHOL HISTORY**

Alcohol is our favourite drug. Most of us use it for enjoyment, but for some, drinking can become a serious problem.

Let us discuss 'sensible drinking'?

It is a good idea for all of us to keep track of how much we drink. We can do this by counting the number of units we drink in a week.

A unit is the amount of alcohol found in half a pint of beer, lager or cider; a short of whisky or other spirits; and a small glass of wine or sherry.

If you drink less than 21 units a week for a man or 14 for a woman, you probably will not have a problem – as long as you spread it out across the week.

Give yourself at least two alcohol-free days each week. It is wise not to drink more than 2 units in any one day for a woman and more than 3 units in any one day for a man.

We all tend to underestimate the amount we drink. One way of finding out exactly how much we are drinking, is to keep a diary for a week, writing down each day how much we have had to drink. If we do this every now and then we can check how much alcohol we are actually drinking by adding up our score in units.

Alcohol can cause physical health problems, mental health problems and social problems.

How can it affect our physical health?

Being very drunk can lead to severe hangovers, and can cause tears on the food pipe resulting in massive bleeding, vomiting blood, unconsciousness and even death.

Alcohol irritates the stomach walls and can cause gastritis. It can make stomach ulcers worse. Drinking too much over a long period of time can cause liver disease and increases the risk of some kinds of cancer.

How can it affect the liver?

The liver has to work hard to get the alcohol out of the body. After a certain period the liver becomes exhausted and it starts failing. This can cause hepatitis and jaundice. After some time it starts shrinking, causing cirrhosis of the liver which kills the person.

What else can it do to our body?

In fact, alcohol affects every system in the body. It can damage the pancreas and interfere with blood glucose. Alcohol can cause heart problems.

Alcohol is the commonest cause for people ending up in casualty with broken bones or head injury. Alcohol is a very common cause of premature death.

Can alcohol affect our mental health?

Excess drinking itself is a mental heath problem. Alcohol relaxes, but only within a certain limit. Beyond that, it causes problems. Alcohol is a very common cause of depression, anxiety and sleep problems. Many people who take overdoses and kill themselves have an alcohol problem and they do so whilst drunk.

In fact, alcohol causes all sorts of sexual problems including loss of erection. In some people alcohol can cause them to hear imaginary voices. This is usually a very unpleasant experience and can be hard to get rid of.

Alcohol can stop your memory from working properly and in extreme cases cause brain damage.

In what ways can it affect our brain?

Alcohol is toxic to the brain cells. When people drink too much for too long, the nerve cells are affected and they can die off. This can cause memory loss and dementia.

Alcohol also affects the nerves outside the brain, for example in the legs and arms. This affects the sensations in our body which we call peripheral neuropathy.

What else can it do to people?

Many problems are caused by people having too much to drink at the wrong place or time. They include: fights, arguments, money troubles, family upsets, and spur-of-the-moment casual sex.

Alcohol is a very common reason for domestic violence and family break-ups. Often alcohol becomes the most expensive thing in people's lives. Many people get into serious debt because of their drinking.

Alcohol can make you do things you would not normally do. Excessive drinking can cause accidents at home, on the roads, in the water and on playing fields.

Sometimes people get into trouble and are convicted for drunken driving or drunk and disorderly behaviour.

What are the warning signs of excessive drinking?

Alcohol is addictive. It is a bad sign if you find you are able to hold a lot of drink without getting drunk. You know you are hooked if you do not feel right without a drink, or need a drink to start the day.

How can I change the habit of excessive drinking?

I am really pleased that you have asked this question. We all find it hard to change a habit, particularly one that plays such a large part in our lives. There are three steps to dealing with the problem:

1. Realising and accepting that there is a problem.

2. Getting help to break the habit.

3. Keeping going once you have begun to make changes.

We can help you to deal with alcohol problems.

What sort of help is available to deal with alcohol problems?

- Initially it may be enough to keep a diary of your drinking and then to cut down if you find you have been drinking too much.

- It helps if you can talk your plans over with a friend or relative. Do not be ashamed to do that. Most real friends will be pleased to help and you may find they have been worried about you for some time.

Getting help

- If you find it hard to change your drinking habits then try talking to your GP or go for advice to a counsel on alcohol.

- Your GP can refer you to the Local Drug and Alcohol Team.

- If you still find it very difficult to change then you may need specialist help.

- Groups where you meet other people with similar problems can often be very helpful. Groups may be self-help like Alcoholics Anonymous, or arranged by an alcohol treatment unit.

- For some people, a short time in an alcohol treatment unit might be helpful.

Are there any drugs available to treat this problem?

If you feel you cannot stop because you get too shaky or restless and jumpy, then your doctor can often help with some medication for a short time.

Drugs are not used very often except at first for 'drying out' (also as 'detoxification'). It is important to avoid relying on tranquillisers as an alternative.

Although beating a drink problem may be hard at first, most people manage it in the end and are able to lead a normal life.

- **Note: It is worth mentioning about information leaflets and fact sheets at the end of the consultation.**

TELEPHONE ADVICE ABOUT A
CONFUSED PATIENT

Task: You are the psychiatric senior house officer on call and you are contacted by the surgical senior house officer on call. He contacted you regarding a 52-year-old gentleman who fractured his leg the day before and underwent major orthopaedic surgery. Today, however, the patient has become very confused, restless, sweaty, shaky and appeared very anxious. The surgical SHO gave a history that the patient is a chronic alcoholic and has been drinking up to three bottles of whisky a day. He seems to have had no alcohol since admission. The surgical SHO is concerned and has contacted you for further advice over the phone.

A. Introduce yourself to your colleague

B. Explore more history which includes:

- Circumstances of the injury and admission

- Past psychiatric history and medications

- Medical history and medications

- Drug and alcohol history

- Current social situation

C. Give priority to alcohol history

- Current usage and longitudinal history.

- Enquire for features of dependence syndrome.

- Enquire about withdrawal symptoms – both physical and psychological symptoms.

- Ask for symptoms of delirium tremens – which include clouding of consciousness, disorientation in time and place, poor attention span, visual hallucinations and illusions which are often vivid and frightening. Tactile hallucinations of insects crawling over body may occur.

- Ask for any autonomic disturbance which include fever, sweating, tachycardia, hypertension, pupillary dilatation.

- Ask about neurological signs and symptoms.

D. Ask about their current management plan and what their team feels about the patient

Ask for necessary blood investigations and other investigations to rule out acute confusional state (FBC, ESR, blood culture, LFT, U&E, creatinine, TFT, chest X-ray, ECG, urine C&S).

E. Give further management advice that includes

1. Safe environment, providing adequate nutrition and nursing support.

2. Nursing in well-lit room and help with orientation.

3. Librium sliding scale (detoxification regime with chlordiazepoxide (Librium) in a reducing dose).

4. Using parenteral benzodiazepines to achieve quick sedation.

5. Maintaining adequate hydration.

6. Instituting parenteral, high potency vitamins (thiamine supplementation or multivitamins).

7. Avoiding use of phenothiazine antipsychotics (haloperidol) due to risk of inducing seizures.

8. Treatment of concurrent infection (if any).

9. Warn about the risk of withdrawal seizures and Wernicke's encephalopathy.

10. Offer to see patient if necessary.

DEMENTIA – COLLATERAL HISTORY

Task: You are in the memory clinic and you have been asked to assess Mr Smith, an 82-year-old gentleman who suffers from memory problems. However, you want to get more information about him from Mrs Smith. Obtain a collateral history from Mrs Smith.

The important areas to be covered are:

- Mode of onset, duration and progression of the symptoms
- Ask in detail about cognitive, behavioural, psychological, physical and biological symptoms
- Risk assessment
- Past medical history
- Past psychiatric history
- Relevant personal history
- Relevant family history.

Suggested approach

- Greet and introduce yourself
- Purpose of visit should be explained
- Obtain permission before you proceed
- Address her main concerns
- Allow her to speak freely for the first few moments noting her concerns
- Start with open questions.

- **Introduce yourself to the patient's relative and address the main concerns**
  a. Please describe for me the problems your husband has been having?
  b. Can you give me examples of his forgetfulness?
  c. Anything else you are concerned about?

- **Onset and progression**
  a. Inquire about the onset of these symptoms, were they sudden or gradual?
  b. Differentiate between sudden onset and sudden recognition
  c. What symptoms were noticed first?

d. When were the symptoms noticed first?

e. How have the symptoms progressed, e.g. slowly progressive versus step-wise?

f. Are there any fluctuations?

1. Cognitive symptoms

Inquire about symptoms in all cognitive domains

Memory – short- and long-term

a. Can he remember things that happened in the last few minutes or in the day?

b. Can he remember events that happened a few years ago?

c. Does prompting or recognition help?

d. Is it consistent or patchy?

Temporal disorientation
Does he know the time of the day, the day of the week, date of the month etc?

Spatial disorientation
How often does he lose his way at home or in the neighbourhood?

Language difficulties

- How about the way he speaks?
- Does he have any word-finding problems?

Comprehension
Can he understand when someone speaks to him?

Dyspraxia

- Does he have difficulty doing things?
- The memory problems that you describe, do they affect his ability to look after himself, or to do the things he used to?
- Inquire about ADL (activities of daily living) skills like maintaining personal hygiene, washing, cooking, laundry etc.

Dyslexia, dysgraphia
What about reading and writing?

Visuospatial difficulties, agnosias

- Does he have difficulty recognising things, places or people?
- Does he have difficulty in recognising familiar faces?

Judgement, decision making

What about planning, making decisions etc?

2. Behavioural symptoms

- Has there been any change in his behaviour?

- Ask about becoming aggressive, violent outbursts, behaving inappropriately, socially withdrawn, wandering at night-time, disinhibited behaviour, repetitive behaviours etc.

3. Psychological symptoms

Inquire about symptoms of depression, apathy, anxiety, paranoia, psychotic symptoms, auditory and visual hallucinations.

4. Physical symptoms

Ask briefly about:

- Sensory impairment

- Weakness of limbs

- Gait disturbance

- Parkinson's disease – any abnormal movements

- Incontinence.

5. Biological symptoms

Inquire about:

- Sleep disturbance and symptoms getting worse at night

- Appetite disturbance

- Loss of weight.

Risk assessment

- Fire risk – safety in the home, cooker etc.

- Management of finances

- Inappropriate use of medication

- Risk of driving.

Other relevant factors in the patient's history

- Current medication

- Past medical history
    a. High blood pressure
    b. Diabetes
    c. Thyroid disorders
    d. Infections
    e. Stroke
- Past psychiatric history: particularly depression
- Family history of dementia
- Risk factors for dementia
    a. Alcohol
    b. Head injury
- Personal history
    a. Education
    b. Occupation
    c. Living situation

- Thank the relatives for their help.
- Explain that we need to assess him further and would like to perform some memory tests, blood tests and a brain scan.

Note: It is almost impossible to cover all the questions in 7 minutes, but it is a good idea to ask at least three or four questions, in each subheading, to cover the important aspects and obtain a global pass!

ASSESS CAPACITY FOR INSIGHT

Task: Mr White is a school teacher admitted to a general surgical ward in your hospital for acute abdominal pain. He had an ultrasound scan for abdominal pain. The scan picked up an appendicular mass, probably appendicular abscess. The surgeons have confirmed that there is a high risk of rupture of the abscess and suggested surgical removal of the abscess.

After the routine work-up and investigations, he has declined to go ahead with the operation, and he wishes to leave the hospital. The surgeons have asked you for advice as to whether he can go, given he has already signed the consent form.

The patient is worried that you will section him so that they can proceed with the operation.

Assess his capacity for insight and address his concern about being sectioned.

Procedure

In order to have the capacity to give consent to treatment, an individual must be able to understand:

- The nature of the problem and proposed treatment
- Why someone has said that he/she needs it
- The treatment's principle risks and benefits
- The consequences of not receiving the proposed treatment.

Also explore:

1. Patient's ability to retain this information and make a reasoned decision
2. Patient's reasons for refusing treatment.

Suggested approach

- Greet and introduce yourself
- Purpose of visit should be explained
- Obtain permission before you proceed
- Address his/her main concerns
- Start with open questions
- DO NOT TAKE HISTORY

1. The nature of the problem and proposed treatment

- Tell me what you understand about the nature of the problem in your tummy?

- Tell me what is your understanding about the treatment that has been planned?

2. Why has someone said that he needs it?

- Why do you think that you need an operation?
- Why do the surgeons think that you need an operation?

3 & 4. The treatment's principle risks and benefits and the consequences of not receiving the proposed treatment

The patient's understanding of the risks of the procedure

- Have you been told about the risks of having the operation?
- Do you think that it might be painful/you may die?

The patient's understanding of the risks of not having the procedure

- What do you think will happen to this swelling in the future?
- Do you think that you will get better if nothing is done?
- Can you tell me the pros and cons of the operation?

Note: If the patient does not understand the relevant information then ask again and give the information in simple, clear terms and then assess whether he had understood it.

Does the patient believe the above information?

1. Do you believe there is a problem in your tummy?
2. Do you believe that if the swelling is not operated on, it may burst and cause major problems and that you could even die?

Ascertain the final decision

Tell me why you have decided to refuse the operation?

Rule out psychotic symptoms/mood symptoms and ask for any disturbance in thinking or having any unusual experiences

- Assess if the patient has been attentive throughout the interview, could understand and believe the relevant information.
- If the patient has the capacity to make the decision, explain to the patient what you have decided and express your concern that the patient had not made the best possible decision (if the patient still refuses to have the operation).

Address the patient's concern about being sectioned

Explain to the patient that the Mental Health Act (1983) is to ensure the safety, protection and treatment of people with mental illness and that we can section someone only for treatment of mental health problems. Explain that the patient is not mentally ill and that he is not sectionable at the moment (if there is no evidence of mental illness).

- Suggest to the patient that it is important to fix an appointment with the surgeon, anaesthetist and the staff in the ward to discuss the issue again in the near future.

- Explain that the surgical team will ask the patient to sign a 'discharge against medical advice' form which reflects the fact that, although the patient is free to make the decision, it is contrary to the advice of the medical and surgical team.

■ Note: Candidate should offer to come back and reassess the patient at a later time/date to establish 'consistency of thinking and decision making'.

■ Thank the patient and the examiner.

MENTAL STATE EXAMINATION

Task: Mr White presented to the A&E in a confused state and complained of hearing voices. Do a mental state examination for this gentleman.

The Mental State Examination is designed to obtain information about specific aspects of the individual's mental experiences at the time of the interview.

Note: There is no need to comment about behaviour and speech in this station.

Most of the candidates tend to forget to assess cognitive state and insight which also carry equal credit in marks as that of mood, thoughts and perception. If we miss them, it might affect the global rating in that station. So it is very important to cover all the aspects rather than wasting too much time on one particular aspect such as thoughts or perception.

Remember the following order

- Appearance and behaviour
- Speech
- Mood
- Thought
- Delusions
- Perception
- Cognition
- Insight

Suggested approach

- Greet and introduce yourself
- Purpose of visit should be explained
- Obtain permission before you proceed
- Build rapport and address the patient's main concerns first
- Explore the main concerns. If not, enquire about his mood and take it from there.

Mood

- Enquire about how the patient feels
- Tell the patients to rate his/her mood
- If I were to ask you to rate your mood, on a scale of '0' to '10', where '0' is the rock bottom of how you feel and '10' is the best of your spirits, where would you place your mood over the last couple of weeks?

- Enquire about depressed mood, depressed negative thoughts and suicidal tendencies
- Enquire about expansive mood
- Enquire about autonomic anxiety.

If the patient says, YES to any of these questions, then explore further.

Thoughts

Explore thought content.

- Can you think clearly or is there any interference with your thoughts?
- Are you in full control of your thoughts?
- Do you feel that your thoughts are private (or) are they accessible to others in any way?
- Can anyone read your thoughts?
- Are thoughts put into your head which you know are not your own?
- Could someone take your thoughts out of your head and would that leave your mind empty or blank?

If the patient says yes to any of these questions explore this and ask for an example?

Delusions

Explore the different types of delusions (important and common ones first).

Delusions of control or passivity

- Is there anyone trying to control you?
- Do you feel under the control of some force or power other than yourself as though you are a robot or a zombie without a will of your own?

Delusions of persecution

- How well have you been getting on with people?
- Is anyone trying to harm, or interfere with you?
- Is anyone deliberately trying to poison you (or) to kill you? (or) make your life miserable?

Delusions of reference

- Do people seem to drop hints about you or say things with a special meaning?
- Do you see any reference to yourself on TV or in the newspapers?

Delusions of grandiosity

- Do you have any special powers or abilities?
- Is there a special mission to your life?
- Are you a prominent person (or) related to someone prominent like royalty?

Delusional mood

- Do you ever get the feeling that something odd is going on that you can't explain? (Do familiar surroundings seem strange?)

Pick up the clues from what the patient says and explore further.
Always check whether the delusion is:

Primary or secondary

- How did it come into your mind that this was the explanation?
- Did it happen suddenly?
- How did it begin?

Conviction, explanation, effects, coping

- Even when you seemed to be most convinced, do you really feel in the back of your mind that it might well not be true, that it might be your imagination?
- Do not be satisfied with a 'Yes' answer.
- Probe, elaborate and clarify. Ask who is doing it, why are they doing it, why should they do it and ask how does he know that this is the explanation?
- Ask how he copes, what he has done and what he intents to do about it.

When investigating thoughts, also enquire about:

- Obsessions, phobia
- Preoccupations
- Others.

Perception

Opening question for hallucinations.

Auditory hallucinations

- I would like to ask you a routine question we ask of everybody? Is that all right?

- Do you ever seem to hear voices or noises when there is nobody about you and nothing else to explain it?
- Are voices in your mind or can you hear them through your ears?

A. Second person

- Do they speak directly to you?
- Do they give you orders?
- What do they ask you to do?
- Do you obey?
- Can you carry on a two-way conversation with the voice?

B. Third person

- Do you hear several voices talking about you?
- Do they refer to you as 'he' (or) 'she'?
- Do they seem to comment on what you are thinking or reading or doing?

Visual hallucinations

- Have you had visions, or seen things that other people could not see?
- With your eyes or in your mind?
- Were you half asleep at that time?

Other hallucinations

- Is there anything unusual about the way things feel, taste or smell?
- Does your body function normally?

Illusion

- Did the vision seem to arise out of a pattern on the wallpaper or a shadow?

Ask about other perceptual disturbances (derealisation; depersonalisation).

Sensorium and cognition

Level of consciousness

A. Orientation

- Time (day, date, year, time of the day)
- Place (name of the place/hospital/floor)
- Person.

B. Attention and concentration

- Subtracting serials of 7s from 100

C. Memory

- Working – immediate
- Digit span 6 plus or minus 1
- **Short-term memory:**

  Name and address: immediate and 5 minute recall
- **Long-term memory:**

  Personal events:

  a. When did you get married?

  b. When did you finish school?

  General events:

  a. Who is the prime minister of the UK?

  b. Has anything important happened in the world recently?

Insight

Extent of individual's awareness of problem.

- Do you think there is anything the matter with you?
- What do you think it is?
- Could it be a nervous condition?
- Do you think that the symptoms were part of your nervous condition?
- Thank the patient and the examiner

DISCHARGE ARRANGEMENTS

Task: Mr Taylor is a 34-year-old gentleman with treatment resistant schizophrenia who has recently been commenced on clozapine. His mental state is now stable and he is compliant with medications at the moment. He lives alone. He has no contact with his parents and other family members. He has two or three supportive friends that live nearby.

His discharge package is:

1. Review by the consultant one week following discharge and regularly thereafter.
2. He will be seen by a CPN fortnightly.
3. He has a social worker to help him with his transition to his own flat.
4. He is attending the clozapine clinic and the blood tests are to be done once a week.
5. He has been referred to the occupational therapy department to look at structured activities.

Explain the discharge arrangements with him, establish rapport and approach empathetically.

A. Discuss the issue of discharge, framing it in a positive way

B. Explain clearly the nature and purpose of:

1. Medical review

2. Community psychiatric nurse (CPN)

3. Social worker

4. Clozapine clinic

5. Occupational therapist.

C. Stress the importance of follow-up in terms of relapse prevention

D. Explain the problems associated with stopping clozapine suddenly

E. Explain the importance of weekly blood monitoring and that it will be fortnightly after 18 weeks.

Possible questions that can be asked by the patient:

Who is a community psychiatric nurse?

These nurses work outside hospitals, usually visiting patients in their own homes, outpatient departments or family doctors surgeries, so are called community psychiatric nurses.

How can a social worker help me?

Social workers are employed by the local authority and they are able to help with financial and housing problems.

What is the role of an occupational therapist?

Occupational therapists have special skills in helping patients regain their self-confidence through structured activities and group-work.

Can you tell me more about the clozapine clinic, please?

Before clozapine is started, a blood test is carried out to check that your white cell count is satisfactory (as has happened with you). When treatment starts you will be monitored. The Clozapine Patient Monitoring Service (CPMS) organises the monitoring.

Regular blood testing is the main form of monitoring. You will have a blood test every week for at least eighteen weeks. All your blood results will be reviewed, and, if all is well, testing may change to every second week until the end of the first year of treatment.

The risk of fall in white cell count decreases after the first year of treatment, so if your blood tests have been satisfactory you should be able to transfer to testing every four weeks. Testing will then continue every four weeks for as long as you are taking clozapine.

Important points to be discussed in the review

1. Take the medication as directed by the doctor.

2. Never stop taking your medication without telling your doctor as this can lead to return of your symptoms or epileptic fits.

3. If you think you have a cold, sore throat or any other infection tell your doctor or nurse immediately. They will arrange a blood test to check your white cell count. If your white cell count is normal, you should be able to continue with your treatment, but they will tell you if this is the case.

■ Ensure that patient knows exactly who they are seeing, and when they are seeing them.

■ Give the patient an opportunity to ask questions.

VALPROATE SEMISODIUM

Task: Mr Black is a 32-year-old gentleman who is an inpatient in your ward and suffers a manic episode. He has a lengthy history of bipolar affective disorder with recurrent episodes in the past. He has been tried on other mood stabilisers without much benefit. Your consultant has decided to start him on valproate semisodium (Depakote). Explain the drug to the patient and address his main concerns.

For what is valproate used?

Valproate is generally used in the treatment of epilepsy to help control fits or seizures. Valproate can also be used to help mood disorders (especially if the person is high – as an antimanic) and some other illnesses, particularly when other treatments have not been effective.

How does valproate work?

It is not entirely clear how valproate works (either as a mood stabiliser or as an anticonvulsant), as it causes several actions in the brain. There is a chemical messenger (or 'neurotransmitter') called GABA which calms the brain down. In some people, it is thought that there may not be enough GABA in the brain. This lack seems to 'trigger' fits or overactivity/mania. Valproate helps to stop the breakdown of GABA and so leaves enough in the brain thereby controlling overactivity/mania and acts as a mood stabiliser.

How long will valproate take to work?

Valproate should begin to work soon after you start taking it. It may, however, take time before your doctor finds the dose that is right for you. The aim is to achieve a level of medicine in your blood that is high enough to control overactivity, but low enough to cause the least amount of side effects. If you are taking it to help prevent mood swings, it may take several months to reach maximum effect.

Will I need blood tests?

For the first six months of treatment you will need a regular blood test (e.g. every month) to check that the drug is not affecting your liver.

You may then need to have blood tests from time to time to ensure that the dose of valproate is enough and not too much or too little to control the condition for which it has been prescribed.

For how long will I need to keep taking valproate?

This is very difficult to say as people's responses are different. What I can say is valproate is a 'preventative medicine' and you may need to take it for a long time, several months or even years.

What will happen if I stop taking it suddenly?

Never stop taking this medication suddenly or without advice from your doctor, as this may cause an increase in your fits or your symptoms may worsen. When the time comes to stop your valproate, this is usually by a slight reduction in your dose every few weeks.

What sort of side effects might occur?

Like other drugs, it may cause side effects. Some are relatively mild and occur during the initial adjustment period. These can happen in the first few weeks after starting the treatment. They can be unpleasant but often disappear or get better with time. Some people may experience no adverse effects at all. Some of the common side effects are drowsiness, feeling sick, increased appetite, weight gain, you may have an upset stomach and you may feel tired all the time. Some people also complain of hair loss, disturbed menstrual periods in women and on higher doses some patients feel unsteady on their feet.

Will valproate make me drowsy?

You may feel sleepy when you first start taking this drug, so you must take extra care if you are allowed to drive or when operating any type of machinery. This effect should wear off after you have been taking it for a while.

Will valproate cause weight gain?

Valproate can make some people feel hungry and they may put on weight. A few people may put on weight without eating more. If you start to experience weight gain or have other weight-related problems, your doctor can arrange for you to see a dietician for advice.

Will valproate affect my sex life?

Drugs can affect desire (libido), arousal (erection), and orgasmic ability. Valproate has not been reported to have a major adverse effect on these three stages. However, if this does seem to happen, you should discuss it with your doctor, as a change in dose may help minimise any problem.

Can I drink alcohol while I take valproate?

There is no complete ban on drinking alcohol if you are taking valproate, but make sure you do not have more than one or two drinks a day, as it may make you feel sleepier. This is particularly important if you are allowed to drive or operate machinery, and you must seek advice on this.

Are there any foods, or drinks that I should avoid?

You should have no problems with any food or drink apart from alcohol.

If I am taking a contraceptive pill, will this be affected?

It is not thought that the contraceptive pill is affected by valproate.

Can I drive while taking valproate?

If you are allowed to drive, remember that valproate can make you drowsy when you first start taking it, so extra care should be taken when driving or operating any type of machinery. It is advisable to let your insurance company know if you are taking this drug. If you do not and you have an accident, it could affect your insurance cover.

- Ask whether the patient has any more questions
- Thank the patient and the examiner

ALL THE BEST

REFERENCES

Internet sources:

- www.rcpsych.ac.uk
- www.trickcyclists.co.uk
- www.superego-cafe.com

Resources:

- Shorter Oxford Textbook of Psychiatry – 4th edition – Michael Gelder/Richard Mayor/Philip Cowen
- The Maudsley Handbook of Practical Psychiatry
- Management of mental disorders – Gavin Andrews/Rachel Jenkins
- ICD-10 Classification of mental and behavioural disorders
- The Maudsley Prescribing Guidelines – 2003 (7th edition)
- British National Formulary – 2003 (43)
- Present state examination (9) – WING